I0486318

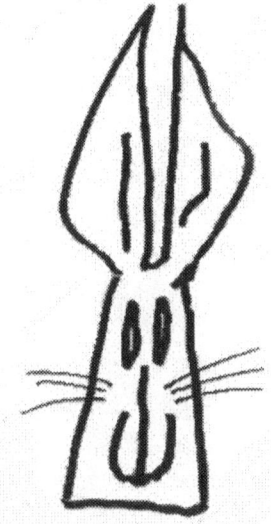

STRANGER IN THE MIRROR

A True Story of Stroke Survival and
Transformation written with Insight,
Compassion and Humor for Brain Injury
Survivors and Their Families

WRITTEN BY

MICHAEL EDWARD LITTLE

authorHOUSE™

1663 LIBERTY DRIVE, SUITE 200
BLOOMINGTON, INDIANA 47403
(800) 839-8640
WWW.AUTHORHOUSE.COM

AuthorHouse™
1663 Liberty Drive, Suite 200
Bloomington, IN 47403
www.authorhouse.com
Phone: 1-800-839-8640

AuthorHouse™ UK Ltd.
500 Avebury Boulevard
Central Milton Keynes, MK9 2BE
www.authorhouse.co.uk
Phone: 08001974150

This book is a work of non-fiction. Unless otherwise noted, the author
and the publisher make no explicit guarantees as to the accuracy of

© 2006 Michael Edward Little. All rights reserved.

No part of this book may be reproduced, stored in a retrieval system, or
transmitted by any means without the written permission of the author.

First published by AuthorHouse 2/10/2006

SBN: 1-4259-0726-1 (sc)

Printed in the United States of America
Bloomington, Indiana

This book is printed on acid-free paper.

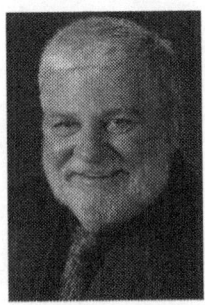

The author looking confident before brain hemorrhage.
If he only knew what lay ahead.

CONTENTS

FOREWORD

Howdy. On May 23rd, 2004, I had a devastating brain hemorrhage while I was reading. An artery supplying my brain with fresh blood suddenly burst and damaged my brain. Stroke is the leading cause of brain damage in America. This book is about my stroke experience, my rehabilitation, and what others should know about stroke. First, I'd like to dispel a popular misconception; stroke isn't the result of over-heated emotions or psychological pressure. In fact, most strokes occur while the recipient is sleeping or otherwise relaxed. I say recipient instead of victim purposely. I don't feel like a victim, or think of myself that way. Victims are those whiny bastards boo-hooing on TV. "Oh pitiful me!" I absolutely refuse to join that crowd. I am a stroke survivor. Period.

Stroke is surprisingly common, but difficult to recognize, because the symptoms can be subtle. If you suspect someone is having a stroke, here are three[1] simple things you can do to find out:

- First, ask them to smile because facial weakness is common to stroke. If they can only manage a broken approximation, that's bad.

- Second, ask them to raise both their arms because limb weakness seems ubiquitous to stroke.

- Third, ask them to speak a complete sentence. Most strokees have speech problems and slurred speech. When I had a stroke, I had all these symptoms. If someone fails to pass any of these simple tests call emergency medical services immediately, describe what you observed, and tell them you suspect a stroke. Don't tarry, as speed is essential to save a life and save a brain.

Seven hundred thousand[2] Americans suffered a stroke in 2004. Of these, one hundred sixty seven thousand were fatal. About the same number of Americans died of stroke last year as all the Americans killed in the Viet Nam war. Where is Hanoi Jane now? Admittedly, posing beside a skilled neurosurgeon and a team of dedicated stroke therapists is less dramatic and garners fewer headlines than posing with a grinning North Vietnamese Gun Crew. Phony is as phony does.

Stroke is America's third leading cause of death and our leading cause of long term disability. Every forty five seconds another American is struck down by stroke. The societal impact of stroke in economic terms, and in terms of human suffering, is immense. Stroke cost fifty three point six billion[3] dollars last year in America, much of it paid for by Medicare and Medicaid. Today four point eight million Americans live with stroke damage. Thirty percent of these are permanently disabled. This lost productivity is stunning. Men who smoke increase their risk of brain hemorrhage every time they light up. Smoking more than a pack a day doubles their risk compared with nonsmokers or men who've kicked the habit[4]. Hemorrhagic strokes account for about twelve percent of all strokes. More than a third of these are fatal. I was a heavy smoker before my stroke. It took a stroke to make me stop smoking cigarettes.

Here are the top ten[5] causes of mortality in the U.S. last year. The body count has increased slightly, but the relationships of the various causes are the same today. We hear annual body counts often in the media, but the numbers are pretty meaningless because they're dizzyingly huge and not in any understandable context. When the numbers are placed side by side, the loss to America is understandable and obvious.

1. Heart Disease   700,142 annual deaths
2. Cancer   553,768 annual deaths

3.	Stroke	163,538 annual deaths
4.	Respiratory Disease	123,013 annual deaths
5.	Accidents	101,537 annual deaths
6.	Diabetes	71,372 annual deaths
7.	Pneumonia/Flu	62,034 annual deaths
8.	Suicide	30,622 annual deaths
9.	Homicide	20,308 annual deaths
10.	Alzheimer's	16,619 annual deaths

I began writing this book while still a patient at the VA Medical Center in Minneapolis, Minnesota. My stroke was the worst experience of my life. I felt like I'd been hit in traffic. I was jerked out of my comfort zone so fast it was nightmarish. The suddenness of stroke is a common sentiment among survivors. My life, my perceptions, and my abilities will probably never be "normal" again. Brain damage changes everything. As bad as the experience was, it was probably the best thing that ever happened to me. Through it I gained enlightenment and a powerful new perspective for living.

Before my experience I had no knowledge of stroke. After having one I began studying stroke. I was shocked and disturbed by much of what I learned. Survivors can have personality changes that are seldom an improvement compared to the person they were before their injury. Some stroke survivors have dementia similar to Alzheimer's.

Before my stroke, handicapped people were invisible to me. I didn't understand the impact of serious impairment on people's lives. Years ago one of my sons was struck by lightning. When he told me about it, I thought it would make a good comedy short. I didn't realize a lightening strike can cause brain damage and some of the same impairments as stroke. Now that I'm brain damaged, there's nothing funny about it. I understand. Brain damage is a creepy subject because the human brain is such a mystery. Today enough is known about the brain that impairments can be predicted with a high degree of certainty. Knowing exactly where the brain was injured will often define the types of impairments the survivor will likely face. Hopefully, you can use what I've learned to advantage. Within these pages I tell my story, which you may find entertaining, interesting, and enlightening. I lucked out because I had a crackerjack neurosurgeon at a great hospital waiting in the waiting room. Now there's an image. After brain surgery, I transferred to a terrific Veterans Affairs hospital that specializes in traumatic brain injury rehabilitation. As a U.S. Army veteran, I qualified for admission to their program. I must warn you, the punch line to my story comes on fast, so read carefully, or you'll miss the point. I see it coming now! It's still quite a ways off, but it's on the way.

Parts of my brain died from lack of oxygen. Brain damage is the most catastrophic event many of us will ever experience. It really rattles your cage. I'm talking about life and death, so it's more than just an inconvenience or a problem with your schedule. Anytime fresh supply blood to the brain is stopped, it's called a stroke. Possible causes for stroke include a hemorrhage like mine, or a small blood clot blocks an artery supplying the brain and stops the flow of blood, thereby starving the brain of oxygen.. This type of stroke is called an ischemic (pronounced iss-kem-ik) stroke. Eighty percent [6]of all strokes are ischemic. A hemorrhagic stroke is also called a "bleed" and is relatively rare. A bleed often results in a blood clot forming inside the skull, which puts pressure on the brain, causing more brain damage. The clot must be removed surgically. Ischemic stroke can sometimes be treated with clot busting drugs. The first type of drugs approved for this purpose is Tissue Plasmin ojen Activators (tPA) Other clot busting drugs are now undergoing Phase II and III testing. Desmoreplase is derived from the saliva of vampire bats and breaks down the fibrin holding the clot in place. Generally, there's a three hour window after the stroke in which brain damage may be minimized if appropriate steps are taken. I sustained some brain damage from my stroke, but the damage would have been far worse or fatal had I waited for surgery. I'm relieved my sense of humor wasn't lost. Areas of the brain cut off from supply blood die quickly. Obviously, dead areas of the brain can't do the job they should. Stroke damage can be devastating, incapacitating or mildly impairing, depending on which areas of the brain are damaged and the severity of the damage. Basic abilities we take for granted can be impaired or lost entirely. These include hearing, seeing, walking, talking, drinking, eating, standing, reasoning and basic muscle control. The good news is medical science and drug companies are zeroing in on stroke full bore. This won't help me or other stroke survivors, but it will help future stroke recipients minimize their damage and their degree of impairment. Another treatment showing promise is high oxygen therapy. High oxygen seems to rescue neurons starving for oxygen. CT and MRI imaging are also very helpful and give doctors new tools so they can identify live and dead brain tissue to aid targeted treatment. Work is underway on drugs that may rescue damaged neurons and help the brain rebuild itself. If successful, these may help all survivors.

In Congress, the House of Representatives and the Senate have recognized the devastating societal impact of stroke and approved the Stroke Treatment and Ongoing Prevention Act. Provisions of the bill provide for improved state access to stroke prevention, treatment and rehabilitation information. Included in this measure is a clearinghouse to share best-practices and a program to educate medical professionals so they are better informed. Stroke awareness and understanding changes constantly as new aspects are discovered and new treatments are developed. The more strokes are studied, new and surprising information becomes available. There now appears to be some linkage between strokes and sleep disorders. The connection isn't fully understood, but studies are under way to understand the relationship. I have sleep apnea. I suspected my apnea contributed to my high blood pressure and to my stroke. I'm relieved my suspicion may have merit.

I spent two years with the 1st Infantry Division in Viet Nam, and since 1969, when I returned home, an equally deadly war has been raging quietly here in America. Stroke has gone largely unrecognized by most people. I've seen few Public Service Announcements that told me anything helpful about stroke. Ignorance of stroke seems widespread. Before my stroke, I didn't know why strokes were bad or what the risk factors were. In fact, I didn't even know what a stroke was! It would be impossible to be more uninformed than I was. Where stroke is concerned, knowledge is power. Families can help speed the patient's recovery with understanding and knowledge. Do your loved one justice, do what they deserve. Educate yourself about stroke. You can help your survivor with knowledge.

You can't possibly help them if you don't understand their needs or what has happened to them. Work hard and educate yourself using the resources in this book. You can do it. Don't let the situation overwhelm you. Brain injured people have special needs. If you and I work together, we will address most of those needs. Even experienced nurses need special training if they are going to work with stroke patients.

A problem with brain damage is we survivors often look "normal". It's easy to over-estimate our abilities or dismiss our impairments. If it weren't for the divot on the side of my head, from brain surgery, I'd look pretty normal. A little body filler, like Bondo, would fix me right up cosmetically. There's no way you could know I'm brain damaged just by looking at me. I don't have any paralysis, the most common indicator of brain damage. In many ways, brain damage is a hidden handicap. Just today I walked over to my bank for an explanation of my latest bank statement because I couldn't understand it. I apologized to the friendly bank lady and told her by way of explanation that I was "slow" because I'm brain damaged. I couldn't understand the statement for a valid reason. She thought I was being self-deprecating and said to me, "Oh, you shouldn't talk about yourself like that." I didn't know what to do, show her my craniotomy scar just to prove my point? I didn't want to embarrass her, so I stammered out a goodbye and walked out. Later on, I thought it was sorta funny, but in explaining my stupidity, I told her too much. I'm not ashamed of being brain damaged, but my status is a bona fide one hundred percent fact. Brain damage spooks people and brings on visions of "insanity". The subject may be unpleasant, but I refuse to hide under the porch out of sight. I won't do it. I'm not proud of being brain damaged, nor am I ashamed. It's simply a fact I have to live with. I'm stupid for good reason. My slowness isn't an act. I don't want people thinking I'm being deliberately obtuse, or playing some sort of game. "Yes sir, I really am this stupid." I used to ignore handicapped people because I didn't know how to talk to them, and I felt embarrassed and guilty because I was healthy and able. Now that I'm handicapped too, I go out of my way to befriend them. They're my people! I just don't have a wheel chair for bona fides. Handicapped people need a friendly smile and a cheerful word, just like anyone else. Since my stroke, I'm not reluctant to look at them or speak with them. My acceptance of handicapped people is an acceptance of myself and part of my transformation, a remarkable process that changed my pride to humility and anger to love. I also reprioritized my life as a result of my stroke. Things that used to bother me don't get any reaction from me now, and I'm much more tolerant. Cat crap on the floor? "Oh, did we have an accident?" I usually don't sweat the small stuff now. It's not worth putting energy and time into something that can't be helped.

In the chapter titled Creating A Safe Harbor, I discuss how you can make the survivor's home safer and more therapeutic. I know these things work because I've used many of them. They come from other stroke survivors, therapists, and doctors. There are things you can do to help make the stroke survivor's recovery and return home less stressful. I address some of these in the chapter titled Survivor Psychology. The human brain is the most complex organ known. Only the human nervous system is more complex. When the brain is damaged, all levels of the survivor's personality, behavior and abilities can be affected.

Despite traumatic brain injury, the survivor may still have a meaningful and productive life. We face challenges unimaginable to "normal" people, but with a little help, the stroke survivor can have a rich rewarding life filled with happiness and satisfaction. The survivor may never be their "old self" again. Do not wait for that person to return. Time may restore them to you, as it has restored me somewhat, but this is impossible to predict. Only time will tell. As a family member and friend, you will have to limit your expectations. No stroke survivor becomes smarter as a result of their injury, although they may become wiser. Personal outlook plays a huge roll in terms of recovery and how the survivor chooses to deal with what has happened to them and the challenges they face. The survivor must find a way to do this. They and the family must search for a working accommodation, something everyone can live with. I found one that works for me and my family, but this is unknown territory and there are no road maps, so everyone must stay open, stay flexible, and do the best they can. I searched hard for a positive side to my stroke. This book is one, and I thank God for it. It took me a year and a half to complete. I'm not complaining though. The process of writing this book was very cathartic.

In many ways, my stroke was the best thing that ever happened to me. When other stroke survivors hear this some are shocked, though not always. I've met other stroke survivors who feel the same way. A stroke is not a pleasant experience, and no survivor wants another. I woke up on Queer Street following brain surgery. Trying to reestablish mental connections and abilities I once had was frustrating and hard work. Some I regained, but not all. Nearly every stroke survivor has some impairment. Happy cheery outcomes following stroke are a rarity. Indeed, many stroke stories are tragic. Some survivors are completely paralyzed and cannot move or communicate even their simplest wishes. Can you imagine the terrifying nightmares those people are trapped in? Other survivors don't understand what has happened to them and are lost somewhere within themselves. Too many outcomes are terribly sad. Many survivors have a rich internal life and carefully relive their memories. This may seem sad, but for many of us, it's all we have. Ultimately, we must each play the hand we are dealt and do the best we can. I'm now handicapped. Psychologically, this was very troubling for me to come to terms with. I'm one of millions of handicapped Americans struggling to live with some degree of dignity. I'll never be "normal", unless I have another miracle. I've already had one that saved me from blindness, madness, and suicide, thank God. Is there a limit on miracles in our lives? I don't want to be greedy, but I could certainly use another. I don't enjoy being brain damaged.

Important note: According to my therapists, people can have recovery from brain injury/stroke up to a year and beyond. Everyone and every brain injury are different. There is no absolute timeline. I had no reason to doubt the year time frame when it was given to me ten months ago. For me personally, it's very accurate. Each day brings new clarity in my perceptions and new competencies as I approach the one year mark. This sharpening of abilities and simultaneous subsidence of impairments is wonderful. My gradual emergence is very exciting, as though I'm gradually awakening. I'm much improved since my stroke. The survivor must be patient, work hard, and never give up! I've improved more than I dared dream possible. My mind has cleared and I no longer feel as if I were walking through a fog. This is noticeable to others through improvements in my speech and a sharper grasp of the world around me. For all survivors, there's still hope until you reach the one year mark. And after you do, who knows? Hang on to hope. I've been working on my rehabilitation a few minutes each day since leaving the hospital. My personal approach to therapy is wishful thinking and prayer. It's unorthodox, but it's slowly working, so I'll continue my daily sessions. There is no way I will be satisfied being handicapped as long as there is the hope I can get back to "normal". Neither should you.

I talk with other stroke survivors often, and I've been surprised at how angry many of them are. They can't understand *why* this terrible thing happened to them. It seems so unfair. I met a woman who had a stroke in her sleep and awakened brain damaged after her stroke. I was surprised to learn thirty one to seventy percent of all strokes occurred while the recipient was sleeping[7]. People who've had an ischemic stroke have a high incidence of recurrence. Often people have a series of strokes. This is scary stuff. If you had an ischemic stroke, talk to your doctor about strategies to prevent a recurrence. It now appears that a daily aspirin[8] and blood thinners lower the risk of recurrent stroke. Patricia Neal, the actress who played opposite Gary Cooper in The Fountainhead, had a succession of strokes and ultimately made miraculous recoveries through hard work and determination. Her example should serve as an inspiration to us all.

When dealing with a stroke survivor, if they make a mistake, don't be surprised. They will make many. It's pointless to be upset, or scream at them, because they're "stupid" or "slow", just as it's pointless to yell and scream at that big oak tree in the front yard because it drops its leaves each fall or because it refuses to produce walnuts. Every living thing behaves according to its nature and capabilities. Limit your expectations. Does your loved one make bad decisions or become disoriented and lost on purpose? Of course not. They're doing the best they can. If you're disappointed with them learn to live with it, just as the survivor must learn to live with their impairments. Be happy you're not in their shoes and count your blessings. No matter the impairments, you can always find someone in much worse shape. T. E. Lawrence, a.k.a. Lawrence of Arabia, said Arabs had a saying, "Every man thinks his fleas are camels," meaning everyone thinks his problems are greater than anyone else's and other people's troubles always appear smaller than your own.

No "normal" person can know the pain or sense of loss a stroke survivor feels when they realize their old life, all their dreams, and their old self, are gone forever. Denouement for me came quietly, like a footpad, unbidden and unexpected. Left alone, I felt as if I were standing on the edge of the world. Out there, in the darkness and emptiness before me, was my death, the end of everything that was me, the end of self. As I stared into the darkness and unknown, I strained desperately looking for hope, but I found none. My fear and uncertainty were consuming. I was terrified. As I waited for death, my chief regret was that I had something I needed to do. Years before, when I joined the Army to go to Viet Nam, I left Miss-Right, the woman I loved, at the airport. When I returned to the states the following year, I was posted to a remote army base in Texas. There, I was caught in a monkey trap. A monkey trap is successful because the trapper understands monkey behavior and uses natural monkey behavior against it. To make an actual monkey trap, drill or carve a hole slightly larger than a monkey's hand in the side of a whole coconut. The bait is a small ball of tinfoil slipped through the hole into the coconut. When a monkey happens along foraging for food, he'll pick up the coconut to see if it can be eaten. When he moves the coconut, he'll hear the foil ball roll around inside. Curious, he'll look in the hole, see the shiny foil ball, and want it. Spurred by natural instincts, the monkey will reach in and grab the foil ball. With his hand clutching the ball, it's too large to pass back out the hole in the coconut. The monkey can't get free of the coconut unless he relinquishes what he wants most. The monkey can't climb with the coconut on his wrist. Stuck on the ground, the monkey is easy prey for predators, and many have gone to monkey heaven clutching a small foil ball. I was the monkey in Texas. Miss-Right-Now was the trapper. The bait was as old as time. I thought I had to have it, and when I did, my pride wouldn't let me relinquish it. I betrayed the only woman I ever loved and trusted for a painted face and bleached blond hair. My betrayal was the most despicable thing I've ever done. I broke Miss-Right's heart. In the back of my mind, I planned to apologize one day, but when I had the opportunity years later, I didn't have the guts to face her. I've been a prisoner of my shame and guilt for almost forty years. Now, because of my stroke, I was afraid I'd die before I could apologize and take responsibility for what I'd done. Death and stroke don't give advance notice so we can tidy up our lives before they arrive. I made a promise to God that if He let me live I'd hunt up Miss-Right and apologize for my lack of moral fiber and weak character. So much time has passed that an apology probably wouldn't mean anything, but with this simple act of contrition I hoped to redeem a measure of self-respect, and come closer to being the man I thought I was.

With death staring me in the eye, I said goodbye to my previous life, and to my self. I felt as if I were dissolving, and felt my self slip quietly over the edge into another world without a whimper or word of good bye. The death of self was the most terrifying and painful thing I've ever experienced. Letting go was excruciating, and terrible, but I couldn't stop the process. Here in Dakota and Montana, we'd say I was forced to "cowboy up." This means to be brave and accept things as they are, and not whine about how we wish they were. I hated the experience, but I had no vote. The process seemed natural, just, and inevitable.

I miss my self, my old self. I'm grieving still, for my self that died in the darkness. I don't know how long mourning lasts, but I'm lonely for what died. Later, a very observant doctor friend pointed out that I was showing the same signs of loss and grief as people who are mourning the death of a loved one. When I thought about it, I realized she was right. Everyone experiences[9] denial, isolation, anger, bargaining, depression, and acceptance before they can come to terms with their loss. I wouldn't let myself believe I was as damaged as experts said I was. Then, I felt angry to think I could be so defective, so handicapped. I don't know if my bargain with God kept me alive so that

I might square away my life is why I lived, but I knew I had to keep my end of the deal. Eventually, I accepted my broken condition, the death of self, and the end of my dreams. Today, more than anything, I miss "normal". Brain damage makes me feel isolated. The world seems further away and less immediate.

Certainly I've lost much to my stroke, but I've gained much too. Wishing my stroke didn't happen is pointless. I might just as well wish I were rich as Crosus and movie-star handsome. One fantasy is as good as another. Feeling sorry for myself is equally self-indulgent and pointless, so I refuse to do it.

After my stroke, I'm "slow." Know what I mean? Wink wink, grin. I don't just mean slow, I mean stuuupid. My cognitive abilities are kaput. I'm not as smart as I thought I was. I feel like a cross between the Rain Man and Forest Gump. Everyday is an uphill struggle, and a series of I.Q. tests I fail too often to help my battered self-image. I try not to look like a dope, but I often do anyway, so I stay in the margins. Others might think I'm quiet or shy, but I'm just cautious.

Many of my roommates in hospital were much worse off than me. One roomy was an Iraqi War veteran who'd lost both hands, been blinded and brain damaged, by an insurgent improvised explosive device. His only complaint was that he'd lost the wrist watch his wife had given him. Compared with this valiant young trooper, my brain hemorrhage was a walk in the park. Injuries like his kept things in perspective. Ironically, we both served in the First Infantry Division, but I preceded Jim by forty years. None of the troopers I met complained about their broken condition. In the presence of brave men such as these, my problems were trivial. Several times during my stroke and hospitalization I had to be brave. Courage is something few of us think about, unless we have a serviceman or servicewoman to worry about. I needed all the courage I could muster to survive with my sanity intact. If you have a loved one who's a stroke or traumatic brain injury survivor, he or she has had to be very brave. There were times when I was scared to death, and so terrified, I prayed to God for the strength and courage to face what lay ahead. I'm not religious, but I'm unashamed of asking for God's help.

I discovered a new breed of twisted humor. Yep, stroke humor. My brother asked if I'd water his "garden" while he was at work. I replied in the affirmative. Knowing I got disoriented and lost easily, his instruction was: "If you get lost and don't know where you're at, pull on the hose until you reach the end. That will be this house." he said. Propriety renders my response unprintable. Stroke humor will be big, even though it's politically incorrect. It'll be big because the audience is growing every day. "Stroke survivors, the woods are full of 'em!" Humor can help the survivor cope with their awful reality. It helped me keep things in perspective. Besides, if you can't laugh at yourself, someone else will. Who you gonna laugh at? The only person I laugh at today is me. Survivor resilience is improved by the ability to find humor in tragedy. Suicide by stroke survivors is surprisingly common I'm sorry to say, though just how common and what the numbers are I can't determine. The reality of a survivor's new world can be overwhelming and deeply depressing, particularly if the survivor doesn't face forward and find something positive from their experience. It's tough though, and I'll not BS you and say it isn't. Stroke can cause clinical depression. This, coupled with the survivor's grim reality, can lead to a tragic end. I was just thinking about my roomy complaining because he lost the watch his wife gave him when his hands were blown off. He couldn't see it anyway because he was blinded in the same explosion. I felt he had bigger fish to fry than lost jewelry. He was a nice kid. He had a beautiful three year old son who came to visit him in hospital. I thought it terribly sad that he would never see or hold his boy. His father would always be the crippled man sitting at home in the darkness, waiting.

My stroke experience felt like I was caught in a long slow plane crash. After the plane hit, it took me a year to climb free of the wreckage.

"A planned life is a dead one[10]. You have to be ready for whatever happens to you." In Butte, Montana recently, a hole mysteriously appeared in the street at the intersection of Glory Avenue and Placer Creek Road. The police are still looking into it. Question: What's the difference between roast beef and pea soup? Answer: Anyone can roast beef.

CHAPTER 1
MY STROKE EXPERIENCE

We often think of stroke as an affliction of the aged. I was surprised to learn this isn't always the case. Stroke can visit children as young as thirty days old and adults of any age. My gender is a high risk factor because more men than women have strokes. My age, which was fifty seven, was another high risk factor because older people tend to have more strokes than younger people. My high blood pressure[11] was another risk factor for stroke. Check yours often. Three weeks before my stroke, Blood pressure was one twenty over one sixty. I knew it was high, but I didn't know why high blood pressure was bad. And now, the kiss of death: cigarette smoking is a huge risk factor. Smoking more than a pack a day doubles the risk of brain hemorrhage compared to men who don't smoke or have quit. I smoked two packs of Marlboro every day for forty years. More than one third of hemorrhagic strokes are fatal.[12] Smoking also increases the risk of ischemic stroke. I enjoyed smoking. I was hooked. I'd tried and failed to stop smoking many times. I started smoking at age nineteen, while I was in Viet Nam, so I'd look older. I looked like Oppie, and the only Army trooper still with his milk teeth. Somewhere in the back of my mind I worried a little bit about cancer, but that was as far as I became concerned with my personal health or well-being. I felt I was living a charmed life and didn't have to worry about my health. I survived two years in Viet Nam, was wounded by friendly fire, survived numerous attempts on my life, and laughed off several Texas death threats and two Texas wives. I thought I was bulletproof at age fifty seven, thirty pounds overweight, and a forty cigarette per day habit. As Bugs Bunny might wisecrack, "What a maroon!" I've wised up some since my stroke. This is how it happened.

On May 23rd, 2004, I was reading a Hopalong Cassidy novel by Clarence Mulford, the best western author ever, late at night when an artery on the right side of my brain burst and began bleeding into my skull. I suddenly experienced the mother of all headaches. Headaches for me were rare. I'd had fewer than five in my entire life. As I read, the words on the page broke apart into individual letters that started crawling off the page like ants off a paper plate. It was a hallucination, and it wouldn't be my last. I walked to my bathroom to get some aspirin, the only pain reliever on hand. I felt "removed," very "spacey." I looked in a mirror as I passed by and was shocked by what I saw. My mouth drooped on the left side. Suddenly my bowels knotted up and my stomach did a flip. My face looked like melted wax. I suspected I was having a stroke because of the droop. I remembered seeing Kirk Douglas after his stroke. Following a short bout of diarrhea, I vomited. This worried me because I'd seen many animals let go from both ends when they were fatally injured. My left leg wouldn't work, and my left arm felt like it was made of wood. Walking was impossible. I fell more than a dozen times while returning the thirty plus feet to my bed. Each time I got up, only to fall again. I refused to just lay there. My thinking was confused and clouded, but I vaguely knew I was in trouble. I finally fell between my bed and my clothes closet. I was stuck and couldn't get up because my left arm seemed dead. It felt alien and lifeless. With my right arm I started slamming the sliding closet doors together and finally attracted my brother's attention, who was upstairs watching television. When he came in and asked what the racket was all about, I told him I'd had a stroke and needed help. When he saw my distorted features he went for the phone and called nine one one. Within minutes, an ambulance hauled me to St. Alexius Hospital in Bismarck, North Dakota, just across the Missouri River from my home in Mandan.

Speed is critical in treating stroke. At the hospital, an MRI confirmed a stroke because a fist-sized blood clot had formed inside my skull. I felt drunk, goofy, and I couldn't think straight. As luck would have it, I'd taken my partial plate out for the evening before retiring. In hospital, I was very vocal and jabbered like a drunken idiot. I knew what I wanted to say but my mouth just wouldn't make the sounds I intended. That didn't shut me up though. I sounded like a very drunk Gabby Hayes. "They went thata way, Woy!" Dr. Thomas Spagnolia opened my skull and removed the blood clot from my brain. When I awoke in the recovery room, I thought I was at home and didn't know why nurses were in my room. I wanted a smoke, but when I tried to get up, I discovered I was strapped to my bed. I asked a nurse to set me free but she talked crazy and wouldn't help me. Instantly I flew into a rage and cussed her up one side and down the other, but it didn't help. She wouldn't set me free and I couldn't get free. My fury continued to build as I strained at my bonds and plotted revenge on the women who dared tie me to my bed. I fell asleep, planning to kill them when I awoke. Several hours later, my murderous plans were forgotten and my restraints had been removed while I slept. My head was wrapped in bandages like Claude Rains in "The Mummy" and I felt like Frankenstein, built from spare parts. "Urrgh! Fire ba-a-ad. Friend g-oo-d." I expected townsfolk carrying torches and pitchforks at any second.

Eight days after surgery, I was discharged to the VA Medical Center. Dr. Spagnolia met me as I was leaving and talked to me like a Dutch uncle. He explained the risk factors of stroke. For the first time in my life, I paid attention. I wasn't well, but I was alive.

CHAPTER 2

BAGHDAD ON THE MISSISSIPPI

The eight hour drive from Bismarck to Minneapolis, that fabled Baghdad on the Mississippi, was exhausting. I looked and felt close to death, but I was encouraged somewhat because I'd be seeing the brain wizards the following day. Like the scarecrow of Oz, I was traveling to a distant city to get a functioning brain. Mine wasn't hitting on much. As an intermediary, it wasn't telling me what my senses were reporting. My vision was dark and filled with static. I knew what I was seeing wasn't what was really going on. My hearing was muffled and my world was dark and chaotic, like a gloomy fun-house. Walking was difficult because the ground appeared to ripple as I moved. Simply stepping over a curb or using stairs was a trial, and I couldn't be certain of my next step. I felt like the Coyote in Road Runner cartoons, always about to step off a cliff. Simply walking was difficult because my left leg was rubbery and my pace halting. My left arm was nearly useless and my movements were jerky. Simply thinking was difficult because I couldn't organize my thoughts or focus on anything for long. Try as I might, my thoughts were chaotic and reminiscent of a street brawl.

Early the next morning, June 3rd, 2004, I arrived at the entrance to the VA Medical Center where I walked directly into a large revolving entrance door and smacked into it head first with a loud thud. "I didn't see it coming," I said with a straight face, ignoring the laughs of the onlookers. Just before noon, my brother and I were introduced to Dr. Marilyn Weber, head of the Traumatic Brain Injury Rehabilitation team I was assigned to. My impression was of a strong capable woman who was all business. I liked her razor sharp intelligence and her serious demeanor. I felt safe in the hands of this attractive professional. Next, one of those thin plastic hospital ID "code" bracelets was put on my wrist. Then, a "wander alarm" was put around my wrist next to it. This is something like the electronic anklets prisoners under house arrest must wear. It was roughly the size of a large digital watch and relatively light. I was told it would trigger alarms if I left the ward without permission. The chances of me tolerating a "wander alarm" were pretty thin, given my reaction to being strapped to my bed. Then, I asked my brother to walk me outside before he headed for home so I could grab a smoke. When I finally went up to three eff, my ward, I felt abandoned and hoped my brother wouldn't ditch me in this strange place. Later, when I asked to go outside so I could smoke again, I was told I couldn't leave. I said "Xin Loi." (Vietnamese for "Sorry about that.") and hobbled through the ward door to the main entrance somewhere beyond. Just as I'd been warned, claxons sounded, bells rang, and lights flashed, creating a perfect pandemonium. "Ah-oo-gah! Doctor Moe, doctor Larry, doctor Curly!" Two male nurses chased after me, but they didn't have to run too fast. I was warned I'd be arrested when I got to the lobby. "Yeah right," I answered back, "I just had my brain scrambled! Cops don't mean anything to me!" I said, with all the bravado I could muster, while the goon patrol returned to the ward without me. Now on my own, I got lost immediately and couldn't find my way out of the darned building. A few minutes later, I reluctantly returned to my ward, completely chastened. The VA Medical Center was wonderful and exactly what I needed, but, as I was repeatedly told while I was there, "This isn't a hotel. You'll have to work here, but this is a good hospital." I was blessed the day I slammed into the front door and was admitted. Whatever modesty I may have had I should have left at the front door when I was admitted. Over the coming month I would be poked, prodded and felt up like a prom date after drinking too much Sloe Gin. *"I love the way your eyes sparkle in the moon light."*

My experience with the Veterans Affairs Medical System following my stroke was very positive. I received a level of care that would easily rival any civilian facility. This was a pleasant surprise, because my only previous exposure to the VA Medical System was immediately after my discharge from military service in nineteen seventy at Hines VA Hospital in Chicago. At that time, Hines could best be described as a snake pit. The facility was filthy and manned by an indifferent staff delivering a level of care consistent with any third world backwater. It was shameful. Outside the entrance a crowd of "visitors" hung out. Some of these birds spent time with patients hoping to ingratiate themselves to a veteran and eventually get written into their will. The tools for this confidence game were oily smiles, repeated visits, small gifts, cookies, fresh fruit, get-well cards, pretended concern, and feigned friendship. These guys were con-artists, grifters, and opportunists driven by greed hoping to make an easy score. A friend and neighbor named Swede spent more than a year at Hines undergoing numerous surgeries and struggling to rehabilitate himself after being shot in the head. When Swede finally came home, he had a tribe of grifters attached to him like remora, anxious for a piece of Swede's thousand acre Illinois corn farm or the million dollars it was worth. After some time, the grifter king suggested his sister would make Swede the perfect wife, and promoted her as "The Ginger Rogers type." Swede didn't want a wife. He was brain damaged, not stupid. He definitely didn't want to marry the grifter king's sister, but the king was persistent. After rejecting countless entreaties for almost half a year, Swede finally relented and agreed to meet "Ginger". The king, his wife, and "Ginger" arrived at Swede's farm one sizzling hot August afternoon to find Swede lounging in a lawn chair in the front yard sipping lemonade in the sun. After introductions were made, the "Ginger Rogers type" turned out to be more the "Peg-Leg Pete type", unkempt, unshaven, and goofy. In a bizarre sequence of events Hollywood filmmakers couldn't invent on their best day, Swede accidentally broke the foot off "Ginger's" wooden leg after she fainted from sun-stroke. With "Ginger" unconscious in the back seat of the grifter-mobile, the whole thieving tribe pulled out in a shower of gravel and curses that must have sounded like music to Swede's ears. "Ginger" and the grifter king were never heard from again. Presumably, the tribe found another veteran and easier pickings "somewhere over the rainbow".

A visitor's agenda may include peddling religion, as I discovered. Like other opportunists, they wrap themselves in a false flag of concern, care, and friendship, but seldom the truth. One closet lunatic rubbed up next to me while I was a patient at the VA Medical Center. I wondered at his sudden friendship, and was mildly suspicious of his motives, because I remembered Swede's experience. His stated reason for spending time with me and other injured veterans didn't ring true. He always seemed sort of constipated, like he was holding something back. One day, after more than a year, his halo slipped and his smile dropped. It was like watching my cat turn into a dog. He got angry when I repudiated his fundamentalist views, and accused me of deceiving him. Part and parcel of stroke recovery is the evolution of personality as it gradually emerges and develops a sense of self. He couldn't claim any moral high ground because his entire persona was built on subterfuge, misrepresentation, and a hidden agenda. I was upset, just as I would have been upset had I discovered a "friend" was just a car salesman looking to sell a rolling junkyard to me. These guys are like carnival hucksters peddling miracle knives and waterless carwash with sideshow trickery and misdirection to prevent rubes from discovering their true purpose. If this wasn't the case, they wouldn't go to such lengths to conceal themselves. How these guys hope to make "converts" with lies and deceit is beyond me. I had need for spiritual support while I was in hospital and when I did, I spoke with a legitimate on-site chaplain. Even though I'm not religious, I'm not against religion or religious people, but I am against liars, hypocrites, phonies, and skunks of every stripe. If someone uses underhanded tricks and misrepresentation in the name of God, they'll have some explaining to do if they reach the pearly gates, regardless of their high-minded, lofty intentions. This is the worst sort of intellectual hypocrisy and spiritual deceit. Doing bad to do good? Do they suppose God will overlook their trickery?

One thing I've noticed about these "religious" birds is they dance around the letter of the law like they were dancing around a minefield, careful not to put a foot wrong, but ignore the sprit of the law when it's convenient or gets in their way. These "gray area experts" often justify their flexible morality by reciting their mantra, "I didn't break the law." *"True enough, Roscoe, you just ignored the spirit of the law. Fifty demerits!"* Can I get an Amen?

Some people will twist, distort, and misconstrue what I've said, even though I've tried to make myself plain. It seems as though some people go out of their way to "misinterpret" and misconstrue anything that isn't part of their canned fast-food dogma. To those who deliberately misconstrue, construe you. But, I digress...Sorry for the soap box.

CHAPTER 3
ESCAPE AND EVASION

On my way back to my room, I swiped a pair of scissors off someone's desk and cut the wander alarm off my wrist when I was alone. I still wanted a smoke so badly I had the heebee gee-bees, so I decided to jump the reservation. With my wander alarm palmed, I went to the main desk in the nurses area and swiped a piece of Scotch tape. I used the tape to attach the wander alarm to the bottom of a food service cart parked outside the dining room. I knew if I hid the alarm on the bottom of the cart, it would be impossible to disable. So, when the cart was moved through the ward door back to the cafeteria, all hell would break loose. *He he he.* Sure enough, as I was slipping down the back stairwell to smokers freedom beyond, I heard the alarms sound off and I grinned like a happy idiot. I love it when a plan comes together. My progress was slow because I was nearly blind, as I will explain later. As I slipped down the back stairs, I sang a few airs of a great old Jerry Butler song from the sixties, "Only the Strong

Survive," in my best basso profundo shower voice-o. I'm no singer, but the stairwell echoed like a great shower. I was so happy to be making my getaway, I laughed like a kid. When I got to the bottom of the stairwell, I walked out the steel man-door and into the night, wearing hospital scrubs and a pair of "detox Reeboks." These are light sock-like slippers found in detox units around the world, I'm told. Very fashionable. It was this or my Nacona cowboy boots, Wrangler Jeans, a Panhandle Slim shirt, a hand tooled belt and one of my several Resistol cowboy Hats. I come from Montana and North Dakota. Out here in cow country, this is de rigueur. Après round-up if you will. As a western writer, Montana native and Dakota resident, this was my usual attire. Not particularly appropriate for "sneaky Pete" work, but it was all I had, other than scrubs and the Detox Reeboks. Three or four smokes later, I made my way up to the third floor and back to my room. To say I was gleeful, as the staff chased their tails inside, is an understatement. My laughter was subdued, however, because I was dazed and confused. I didn't know where I was most of the time I was outside. I was horribly disoriented and constantly lost. I had a difficult time just seeing and nothing made much sense. All I knew was that I'd jumped the reservation easily, and my smokes never tasted so good. If I hadn't been so addled and blind, my breakout would have been big fun.

I'd taken escape and evasion courses (E&E) in the army, and I was confident I could keep the staff chasing their tails. The theory behind the E&E courses is a soldier escapes and evades capture behind enemy lines. His first priority is to foul up enemy routine, harass them and destroy their sense of safety, security and normalcy. This is easily done by destroying vehicles and disrupting normal operations. Be a pain in the enemy's hind parts, and undermine morale. I had huge fun with my wandering, but I was operating under a tremendous handicap. My brain was scrambled, my thinking was confused and my vision was terrible. "Attention mister and missus America, and all ships at sea, Mr. Magoo has escaped from the hospital! Be on the lookout for a middle-aged cowboy chain smoking Marlboros. That is all!"

In fact, I was almost totally blind. I discovered the following day I had a "left field cut." The stroke had damaged the vision center in my brain. Because of this, I bump into things, like the revolving front door, that approach from my left. In daily living, I tend to neglect the left side of everything and must scan constantly so I don't miss the left half of the sentence when reading, the left half of the picture when watching television, or the left half of the world. I'll never drive again because of my field cut and neglect. I used to be an avid drag racer and raced for years on various strips. I love speed and racing.

I've spent serious money on fast cars over the years, but I've never gone too fast, or fast enough. Speed and racing were casualties of my stroke. I can still ride horses but must rely on them not to get us into a wreck.

My stroke destroyed other things as well. I used to take pride in my stalking ability, and I've stalked deer to within touching distance. They really jump when they realize I'm beside them. Stalking is easy if you know how to stay within an animal's weaknesses. All it takes is specific knowledge of the animal you intend to stalk, discipline and patience. Every animal has strengths and weakness. If you stay within its weaknesses and stay away from its strengths, anyone can be successfully stalk wild game. It's huge fun and a great test of skills. With my field cut, I can't sneak up on anything because I make too much noise banging into stuff. Acute hearing is a strength for most animals, and the ability to move silently is critical. Victory goes to the bold. I'm not Rambo, but I've gone through jungle school, survival school, and I've hunted deer and bear since I was a kid. I love the outdoors and I'm at home there, particularly at night when I'm in the woods or fields. I'm happiest when I'm up to my chin in nasty. I grew up in the wild and love that element, the more difficult the better. As the song says, "I run through the brambles where a rabbit wouldn't go." It's just a game to me, a game I love to play.

My desire to smoke drove me outside repeatedly. My love of pranks added zest to my forays, and added some enjoyment. I'm also a former martial arts instructor and I've had years of training in various disciplines. The stroke and surgery left me weak as a kitten. I was terribly out of shape physically and mentally. I knew I needed the staff for my rehab, so I didn't harass them too much. As a Veterans hospital, there were lots of guys around like me, trained to raise a lot of sand with soft targets. That's why you don't want to make us angry at petty Mickey Mouse junk or screw with our lives. Particularly when we're trying to stop smoking! Are you reading me nurse M? I haven't forgotten you, big sister. Pull my finger.

During the next several weeks, I was caught outside sans wander alarm many times by the staff . When they asked about it, I'd tell 'em the truth. "I got tired of it and cut it off." "We'll just have to replace it then", a particularly prissy nurse said to me, dripping with self-righteous indignation and officious contempt. In the coming weeks, my wander alarm was replaced with untiring regularity. The day I was discharged, I had a drawer full of wander alarms. I thought of it as my wander alarm collection. Scissors were easy to swipe. I discovered another prank by accident. I found that if I hid out of sight around the corner from a ward entrance, I could trigger all the alarms if I got within fifteen or twenty feet. When no one appeared, it would drive the nurses on the front desk crazy. Hidden around the corner out of sight, I'd listen to them complain about the system and wonder why it was acting up. I laughed 'til I almost cried. My life didn't have much fun in it, so I took my laughs where I could get them. I'm not a guy who used to put a flaming bag of dog poo on someone's doorstep, ring their doorbell, and then watch from the bushes as they stomped out the fire, scattering dog poo in every direction, but it's the same sort of idea.

CHAPTER 4
A DIFFERENT POINT OF VIEW

One afternoon I desperately wanted a smoke and went A.W.O.L again. Outside, I struck up a conversation with a pretty young nurse standing beside me at the bus stop in front of the hospital, where I stood smoking. "This must be a pretty depressing place to work," I said to her casually. "Why do you say that?" she asked. "Well," I replied, looking around at all the walking wounded, "Most of the patients here are wrecks, like me." " I suppose some of them are pretty bad off," she replied with an "I've go a secret" Mona Lisa smile, like she knew something I didn't. I thought she'd lost touch with reality a few clicks back. "Hey, Hotel Goofy is right around the corner. Maybe you should check in," I felt like saying. From where we stood, I could see dozens of people in wheel chairs, pushing IV stands, hobbling around on crutches, mincing along with walkers, and staggering along on canes. With all the injured banging around, the place looked like a train wreck.

"It's not depressing at all. I get to see the recoveries," she said to me. I thought about it, and suddenly it hit me. She was absolutely right! This pretty young nurse taught me a valuable lesson right then. She was in a privileged position to see miracles every day. She got to see life's happy endings, and she felt fortunate for it. How wonderful for her! I now understood her secret smile. The hospital was inspiring to her, not depressing. She loved her job. Where I saw only tragedy and human wreckage hobbling around, this woman saw hope, recovery and rebirth. Wow! She changed my view of hospitals entirely. I soon started looking for the positive side of my stroke, but I couldn't find it. I searched and searched for my own happy ending, but I couldn't find anything in my whole horrible experience. I suspected it must be there, but I just couldn't find it. That young nurse really opened my heart and got me thinking about my viewpoint, and how crippling and limiting it was. I had to be missing something. My blindness truly was crippling, depressing and incapacitating. There was nothing I could do about it, was there? I thought of some bubba saying, *Nope, he's blind as a bat.* It was hard for me to find anything positive about my situation. It seemed so hopeless, and I felt doomed. I was treading water just keeping my sanity, floundering in the unknown. I didn't know how long I could stay afloat. I was paddling as fast as I could, but I seemed to be losing ground. All the exertion was exhausting me.

CHAPTER 5

VOLUNTEERS

The VA Medical Center has the support of a great many volunteers who were a great help to me and other patients in the one thousand plus bed hospital. These wonderful people served as escorts and guides for me and other patients, or they pushed us around if we were wheelchair bound, as I was for a while. This quiet, caring cadre deserves great credit and my eternal thanks. If not for them, I couldn't have completed the rehabilitation program. Disorientation is a common problem for right hemisphere stroke patients. I felt like a lost rat searching for the cheese most of the time in the maze-like corridors of the hospital. Thank God for all the wonderful volunteers! I needed them, and they were a very positive force in my life.

One evening a friendly escort called and said he'd be bringing me some hamburgers and french fries from a local golden-arched fast-food restaurant. I don't remember the name. This was good news I couldn't wait for. Near the time my burger delivery was due, I slipped down to the main entrance to take delivery. When I got to the lobby, I noticed the usual policeman at the information desk was absent. With nearly half an hour on the clock before my burgers were due, I took a seat at the information desk. I thought it would be big fun pretending to be a hospital employee in my scrubs, and it was. I directed visitors to the gift shop, the lab where they could donate blood, the chaplain's office and other destinations. It was a hoot pretending and helping out. Half an hour later my friendly escort arrived and was surprised to see me manning the information booth directing lost lambs. "Hi, what are you doing here?" he asked. "Oh, I'm just helping out," I replied laughing. We quickly retired to the break room and I quietly abrogated my responsibilities in favor of burgers and fries.

When I was stationed in Viet Nam during the war, my company, the 337th RRCo 1st Infantry Division, supported a nearby Vietnamese orphanage. I volunteered to help out with monthly supply runs carrying food, supplies, and medical aide to the children. What I saw at the orphanage was shocking, because many of the children were themselves casualties of the war that had killed their parents. Some were so horribly disfigured from their injuries I wondered what sort of life they could have. I pulled guard duty and perimeter security while medics treated the children and they were fed. While standing on the wire I noticed a beautiful flower bush with bright pink blossoms on the other side of the barbed wire from me. As I admired the beauty of the tropical flowers I noticed one strand of barbed wire bisected one of the flowers perfectly. The juxtaposition of the steely wire and the petal softness of the flower seemed to epitomize the war perfectly. The country and the children were once beautiful but were torn apart by the war. Later, back at base camp, I made a pen and ink sketch of the bisected flower and sent it home to my father. When I finally returned home my mom said my dad cried when he saw my sketch and read the story behind it. I get misty eyed today when I think about it. Helping those children was my first brush with volunteer work. I was a community volunteer for twenty years before my stroke, and was concerned that my brain damage would halt my volunteer efforts, but I was wrong. I returned to volunteer work shortly after I was discharged from hospital. Even though I'm brain damaged, I can still be of value to my community. Before a survivor learns the scope of their impairments, it's natural to experience feelings of worthlessness and uselessness. After the survivor learns their capabilities, they can find a place where they can share their experience and time with people who need it if they are so inclined.

I urge everyone to volunteer to help others if they have the time. Since I began volunteer work, I've been a community activist, a children's literacy mentor in public schools, a Guardian Ad Litem in district court advocating for the rights of children, and a hospice volunteer spending time with dying veterans. Not everything I've done was particularly important, but some of it was. I've had a positive effect on people's lives. No matter what I'm doing, I'm happy to do it. This may seem trivial, but my volunteer activities have brought satisfaction and a sense of accomplishment to my life. My future, which looked so barren and bleak after my stroke, now looks like acres of diamonds.

Forty four percent of all Americans age fifty five and older donate an average of four point four hours per week, totaling five point six billion[13] hours annually. Volunteers are proven[14] to stay active longer and have fewer health problems than non-volunteers, so volunteering is a win-win situation. There are several groups that help organize and coordinate volunteer work. The one I'm involved with is the Retired Seniors Volunteer Program. Another active organization doing good work is Experience Corps. I don't mean to get preachy on you. You either see or feel the need to help out or not. If you don't, that's your business. I'm strong on volunteerism because it builds a strong community and a better world. It's more suited to older citizens though. When I was young and working hard everyday, I didn't have time to spare for volunteer activities or anything beyond my family and their needs. Don't get the idea that I'm a community gadfly with my photograph in every newspaper. In the past ten years my photo has been in the newspaper once, when I was sworn in as a Guardian Ad Litem. I simply want to help out where I'm needed, without any fanfare.

CHAPTER 6
LOST IN THE OZONE

I mentioned several times I was nearly blind after my stroke. This will be difficult to explain and difficult to understand, so please, stick with me. All of us hear those around us complain about how difficult their life is, how heroic they are under the circumstances, or what someone told his wife, or what she said to her husband, or what so and so said to their blankety blank boss. Given this conditioning, It's easy to trivialize other people's torments, but just imagine for a moment, if you can, it was you who was lost in the ozone, not your humble scribe. My stroke occurred on May 23rd, 2004. For the first eight weeks that followed I seemed to have a dark cloud hanging over me. It was so dark it blocked out the sun and cast a deep shadow on everything around me, wherever I went. Everything around me seemed to be in shadow, deeper and darker than normal. I couldn't get enough light to see anything very well. Even in direct sunlight my world was dark, gloomy, colorless, and difficult to make out. My world was just various tones of gray. What I saw was like looking at the world through very dirty windows, or watching a poorly tuned television whose picture is nothing but black and white spots that some people call "snow" or static. It's usually accompanied by an irritating hissing sound. That's all I could see, black and white spots jumping around. The cloud and the static left me nearly blind. I was a fine arts major in college and made my living as a professional designer for nearly thirty years. My eyesight was absolutely crucial to me. Now I couldn't read. I couldn't see the world around me or the pages of a book. It was always too dark, and I couldn't make anything out clearly because of the dancing spots. Concentration was impossible, because the black and white spots jumping around were very distracting. As week followed week, I fell into a deep depression and I thought of suicide constantly. Death seemed preferable to what my world had become. There was no relief, seemingly no end to my private hell. People were silhouettes, two dimensional cutouts moving about in the graying gloom, alive with flickering spots of black, gray, and white. There was no color, just subtle shades of static. The world looked like it was raining gray confetti wherever I looked. I was seemingly trapped in a Georges Seurat petite point painting with all the delicate nuance of color drained from it. My world was dark, dreary and impossible to see or understand. Nothing made sense. Moving cars and traffic, what I could see of it, gave me the willies and made my skin crawl. The world seemed insane. The ozone was permeated with such an oppressive ennui that it just about made me physically ill. That strange terrible world was a puzzle. Try as I might, I couldn't understand how it worked. I didn't know the rules. I felt that if I could solve the puzzle, I could find a way out and live. I was convinced there was a key to it all, but I couldn't find the key. "No aya le yave," as my Mexican friends would say. It was as if everything was in code and I didn't know how to decode it. I was trapped in an awful joke and everyone knew the punch line but me. My world had tilted on its axis and I didn't know how to fix it. I hated every second of that strange, terrible place and I couldn't wait for death. I felt as if all my senses were being jammed, overloaded. I felt like I suspect an autistic might feel. I was disoriented and lost constantly and never had a clue where I was or how I got there. My disorientation was a constant torment. Twice I got lost in the men's room. Two times I left my room to go someplace and when I got back to my ward, I walked into the wrong room and then hopped into the wrong bed! *Well, excuse me, stranger! Sorry to be so friendly!* This sounds funny I suppose, but I sure wasn't having fun. I was relieved no one was home at those "awkward moments". I was ratted out though, and the staff knew I couldn't find my own bed. My cloud was with me since I woke up following brain surgery and I wanted to kill my nurses because they tied me to my bed. I didn't tell anyone about my living nightmare, because what could anyone do? I was afraid what I was experiencing was all there was. My despair never bottomed out. It grew worse day by day and I abandoned any hope of ever escaping. I was stuck. Many times I felt just like the painting by the famous Norwegian expressionist painter Edvard Munch, titled "The Scream". I was immersed in that horrible place for so long, my anguish was killing me. I forgot what reality should be, or could be. I was a captive of that strange colorless world for more than a month. That was all the time needed for me to forget color and what the real world looked like. Before my stroke I'd been an avid reader, but now I could barely read. I couldn't even see the page! My eyes refused to work together and rolled around in my head like two marbles in a saucer. I couldn't see the words through the static. It was awful. I just wanted it to end. One of my therapists in occupational therapy insisted I use the Minneapolis Yellow Pages in the phone book and find the price of a gallon of flat off-white latex paint. It was like trying to read bird entrails to determine the future. *"Hey! They's just guts to me! They don't say nothin'!"* It would be easier to teach a fish to climb a tree than get me to find a phone number in a book I couldn't see. The alphabet barely made sense, all the letters piled on in a confusing jumble. *"I think I see the leg of an R sticking out. Yep, that's the leg of an R, alright. He's on the bottom. I think he's hurt. His leg looks broken!"* All the phone numbers clustered together like horseshoes around the stake. *"The eight and three look like leaners."* Numbers and letters were incomprehensible, no matter what size magnifying glass I used. I wanted to tell my therapist to stuff it, but I wanted to do well, so I held my frustration in check. I was a writer who couldn't read or see the page. What could I do? Resign myself to living in hell? How could I survive there? I couldn't understand how I could possibly paint or draw anymore. I couldn't fish anymore because I couldn't see well enough to cast or tie on a lure. This was tragic stuff for me. I couldn't see to sketch, write, or fish. I'd have to abandon everything I enjoyed. Without art, fishing, and reading, what the hell could I do? I wouldn't be able to cook my own food. I enjoyed cooking relatively complex Italian ragu gravies. Now I couldn't do much of anything, as my daily therapies were showing. I was almost helpless, and I doubted I'd ever function with any kind of competence approaching my former existence. I was totally handicapped, helpless because I was blind. I was devastated. My outlook for the future was bleak to say the least. I suppose all this just sounds like whining, but being trapped in that awful world for more than a month was hellish. It was so dark, so depressing, so utterly hopeless, and so filled with despair that it was far worse than my years in Viet Nam. War was a cakewalk compared to the ozone. I didn't tell anyone about what I was dealing with because I got used to it. This seems impossible, I suppose. Looking at how quickly kidnap victims relate to their kidnappers, it's easy to see that the constructs we create that define our world are very tenuous. The ozone was horrible. I forgot real world colors, like the rich blue of the sky, the vibrant greens of living plants. The riot of life's glorious colors were missing and forgotten. One day at lunch, things just seemed to build up and I felt my head would explode, so I went to see Dr. Kerri Lamberty, a very skilled and capable psychologist on the recovery team. I didn't tell her about the ozone, but just talking with her seemed to relieve my depression somewhat. When I left her office, I felt less despairing. This brief respite was recharge enough to keep me going. Until all this happened, I didn't believe in hell. My only thoughts on the subject were cartoonish pits of fire, horned demons with pitchforks and other nonsense. I couldn't imagine how bad a hell could be. Now that I've seen how awful things can be, the idea of hell is frightening. Dante low-balled us in the Inferno. The actual experience of living in the ozone far outstrips my descriptive abilities.

CHAPTER 7
SAVED BY A MIRACLE

On Wednesday, June 30th 2004, Laura Barrett, a recreational therapist, and I went to the history museum in St. Paul for a short visit. I'd read some Minnesota history about the Great Sioux Uprising and the Metee people just before my stroke, so I had some knowledge of local history. The museum was terrific, but my cloud was still shadowing me. *Good one, huh?* My vision limited what I could see, but I was able to sorta see exhibits on the Metee people. As we walked out into the sunny afternoon from the museum, I felt the warmth of the sun on my face and breathed the fresh air. Laura asked me to find her darned car, to practice my direction finding and figure out where I was. *I know where I am, I'm in hell! I know exactly where I'm at, but as my amigos say, "no aya la puerta." I can't find the door.* Even when I was relaxing, enjoying the day on the "lido" deck, and "off the clock", Laura wasn't. She insisted I perform one more stunt and "just for fun" find her car. Rust never sleeps. Neither does

Satan. My therapists never relaxed for one moment when they could make me perform one more trick. Roll over! Speak! Curses! I secretly suspected my therapists slept in coffins. Transylvania six five thousand, please.

The car was finally found. I think Laura found it, since it was a colorless X-files government Taurus just like Skully and Mulder's. If we'd waited for me to find the car, I'd have waited until all the cars in the lot went home for dinner. The only car remaining would be Laura's. When we finally left the lot, Laura pulled out into traffic and we headed back toward the medical center. I rode shotgun and watched anxiously as the traffic herd stampeded at us. Ben Hur meets NASCAR. Suddenly, it was as if God flipped a switch on the back of my head. My vision cleared, the static vanished and I could see and understand everything in an instant. The black cloud vanished and I could see perfectly well for the first time in more than a month! Brilliant sunlight shown down and everything was glowing in brilliant hues. The world looked like magic. Suddenly my world had color again. It was thrilling and absolutely beautiful! I can't begin to describe how wonderful everything looked. Bright colors looked like glowing candy, good enough to eat. Delicious. "It's a miracle!" I shouted and jumped as if shocked. Bouncing up and down in my seat, "I can see!" I shouted. "All this traffic looks great!" In a flash, my vision cleared and I understood the world for the first time in ages. It was wonderful!

"God shined His light on me!" I shouted excitedly to Laura, bubbling with happiness and laughter. Then I told her what had just happened. "It's a miracle!" I was so relieved to be out of the ozone, the effect on me was a tonic, like an elixir. I never again thought of suicide after I was healed in that instant. I'm not religious, but I felt God touched me that day. I felt truly blessed, and so grateful, words could not express my joy or relief. I told everyone I came in contact with! I bubbled and enthused! Holy Cats, I'm healed! No more ozone! I was trapped in that perfect hell for five weeks. It was someplace I hope I never visit again. It was so awful, I just wanted it to end. My spontaneous healing was not total. I still have a field cut and a list of other impairments, but just being able to see color without the static and the black cloud is a miracle. The world makes sense, and life's fun again, richer than ever before. Can I get an Amen?

As I type this, my computer just warned me it has a memory leak, which seems ironic, because I do too. My spontaneous healing saved my life. Viewed as anything other than a miracle, the fact that I was instantly healed is inexplicable and seems beyond the bounds of science and medicine. Several times I asked my doctors if spontaneous healings were common, because I wanted to know if what

I experienced was usual for stroke survivors. If they'd told me it happened all the time, then my experience wouldn't have been a miracle. None of them would respond though, and their hearing suddenly went bad. What I didn't understand was this; they couldn't answer me. To do so would have been an acknowledgement of God, an area normally the province of radio preachers, tent revivals, and hill William hucksters peddling snake oil, miracle cures, magic waters and salvation. "If you truly believe, put your hand on the radio!" My doctor's refusal to answer me was probably wise, though not helpful.

I had some difficulty explaining to you everything that happened, dear reader. Whenever I broached the subject of my spontaneous healing with my doctors, they backed off fast, like I was a bum asking for spare change and mumbling incoherently about giant rabbits. Their reactions were interesting and even humorous, but brought no enlightenment.

My healing was a reprieve from hell and I felt the hand of God in my life. It reminded me strongly of an experience I had in nineteen seventy five. After a difficult day at work, I wanted to relax when I got home. When I came in, I first sat on my sofa. After a moment, I leaned over backwards and stretched out on my back. I didn't sleep, because I've never been able to sleep on my back. I closed my eyes and just sorta drifted. Suddenly, I had the most remarkable experience of my life. I met God. The encounter shook me to my foundation and changed my life. For the first time, I started thinking of others and how I could help them. Buddhists say the desire that others not suffer is compassion

I've told many people about this experience if I thought it would help them. Unfortunately, language is poor currency for relating matters that transcend normal human experience. I can describe meeting God, using all the language skills at my command, but reading about it isn't the merest shadow of the experience. For centuries, writers have agonized over this problem. [15] "There is an inside to experience, as well as an outside" So, cast the earth free, open your heart, and I'll take you inside. Imagine….

Somehow, I was subtly transported, and in the blink of an eye I was adrift, weightless, floating in a silent black void. I didn't know where I was, but it was like I'd always imagined outer space to be, except there were no stars, planets, comets, or nebulae to see, things I'd always imagined seeing when I was a kid and an avid science fiction fan. I was disappointed by what I didn't see. Space was just, well, empty space. There was nothing, nothing in the darkness, except a tiny mote of light, a pale white blur. It was so tiny and insignificant that I hardly noticed it. Compared to my childhood imaginings, it was less than nothing, like a wisp of lint lying on the floor across a large room, totally irrelevant. My senses told me I was moving through the darkness very fast, but because nothing was visible I had no way to confirm the sensation of movement or gauge my speed. After what seemed like four or five minutes, I realized I was moving toward the wisp, because it gradually grew larger and brighter, as though I were moving closer to it. When, what seemed like ten or fifteen minutes had passed, I could finally see the curiosity plainly and was amazed, because the irrelevant wisp was a brilliant white star hanging in space. My journey had begun so far away, and the star had looked tiny and insignificant in the distance. Now that I was closer, the star was immense. I was looking down on it from above. It shined like a radiant white diamond on the black fabric of space, and seemed brighter than ten thousand suns. My view was breathtaking. The light was so intense that it was painful to look at, and hurt my eyes. I continued moving closer and dropped down level with the star, and then stopped moving altogether and stood before the star, on what felt like solid ground. I was greatly puzzled and a little apprehensive. I didn't know where I was, but I knew it wasn't normal. The light was so brilliant that I squinted and put an arm over my eyes to block out the painful rays. I felt like an egg being candled, or as if I were being X-rayed. I stood revealed, and felt transparent in the light. I grew uncomfortable in the glare and turned away, looking for something to look at other than the searing intensity of the star, but there was nothing to see, just the brilliant star looming at my back. It was so huge, I felt dwarfed near it. I tried to ignore it. I wanted to ignore it, but its size and brilliance demanded my attention. It was insistent, a presence impossible to ignore, like a four hundred pound gorilla at the breakfast table. *"Oh, just ignore it, dear, and drink your juice. Maybe it'll go away."* Try as I might, I couldn't ignore it. Finally, I got brave and decided to investigate. I couldn't tell how close the burning ball of nuclear fire was, but I thought I should have been burned or at least felt its heat. Instead, I felt neither hot nor cold. It was a curiosity I had to investigate, so I steeled myself to look more closely. I narrowed my eyes and then turned to face it for a quick look, just a peek. I was amazed to see, in the center, a man's face in the luminous ball of fire. He didn't look like anyone I knew, or anyone I'd ever seen before. He was clean shaven, with short hair, sorta parted on one side. He was just a regular looking guy. I saw His lips moving, as if He were speaking, but I heard nothing. I knew sound couldn't carry in space, so I wasn't surprised to hear nothing. As I stared into the radiance, I was dazzled by what I saw, and surprisingly, my eyes didn't hurt as they had earlier. The star man was incredible! I felt like I was watching a silent movie of a man talking to the camera. Then, suddenly, I heard a man's voice in my head, but not with my ears. It was as though He were speaking directly to my mind. The voice matched the movements of his mouth, so I knew the voice I heard was that of the man I saw. In a calm, pleasant voice, He spoke to me about my life and asked what I'd done. When I began telling him about myself, He started looking at my memories of my life. Somehow He pulled memories from me I'd forgotten long before. He rummaged through my life as if he were picking through someone's attic, examining my every deed. He showed me sort of a film of each memory as he examined it, so I knew what He was seeing. I watched episodes of my life as he found them. As we watched each memory, I relived each incident. He even examined thoughts I'd had, and showed me a film of each thought so I could understand each one. In this way, we looked at absolutely everything I'd ever done or thought. I was apprehensive about what he might see, and worried He'd discover some particularly embarrassing or private moments in my life. I braced myself for the embarrassment I felt would surely come, but it never did. After my most private thoughts and deeds were examined, I wasn't embarrassed at all. I relaxed and accepted our shared review of my life with surprising equanimity, as though I did this sort of thing every day. He had my complete trust. As we looked at "films" of countless deeds and thoughts, He did something even more amazing. Somehow, with a snap of His fingers, He compressed each film after we watched it, so that each was turned into something like a playing card. After he made a card of a deed or thought, He dropped it onto one of two piles he was making in front of Himself. As the two piles grew, I understood one pile was for "good things", and the other was for "bad things". The "good things" were instances where I'd helped someone or been kind to someone in some way or had good thoughts about someone. "Bad things" were instances when I'd been mean or unkind to someone or had unkind thoughts. Each instance He compressed into a card, and dropped on one of the piles, while I quietly watched the amazing process. I was surprised that my thoughts were as important as my actions. I'd always assumed my thoughts were my own and didn't mean anything, but I was wrong. My "bad thoughts" were dropped on the pile of "bad deeds." As I watched in amazement, I remember being filled with what I can only describe as love, radiating from Him. His love was joyous, wonderful, vitalizing, and heavenly. His love felt good enough to eat, like food from heaven. It seemed sustaining somehow, as if His love had substance. A jubilant feeling of His love filled me, and I vibrated in harmony with it. I was exalted. At some point, I realized

I was talking with God. Instead of being awed or frightened, I felt accepted and safe. It was a comforting, secure feeling to be with Him. I loved Him so much, I almost hurt. I felt as if I were home for the very first time in my life. It was wonderful, like paradise. I realized how much I had missed Him. He knew me as well as I knew myself, and he accepted me as I was, warts and all. I basked in His acceptance, and I loved Him for it, because I knew He was responsible for my feeling of joy, well being and safety. Finally, when my life had been thoroughly examined, He picked up the two piles of cards, held them side by side and compared them. It took Him just an instant to measure the good against the bad. I was breathless, as I waited for His judgment. When He was done, He told me I had more good than bad. I was thrilled and immensely relieved, because I didn't have any idea if I'd been more good or bad. I don't know what I would have done if His judgment had gone the other way. I don't think I could have argued with him. His judgment seemed beyond reproach and absolutely correct, particularly since I was His witness. There could be no dispute. When my judgment was finished I knew, without being told, that it was time for me to leave. Now that I was home at last I didn't want to go. I reveled in the warmth of His love and begged to stay. I felt wonderful with Him. I was completely accepted, like I always wished my father would accept me. "Please don't send me away! Let me stay. Please! It's wonderful!" I begged, I pleaded, I whined like a child, and dug in my heels and clawed at the "ground," desperate for something to hold onto so He couldn't pull me away. I was pitiful, like a disappointed child who didn't want to leave the circus when it's over. Sadly, God refused my entreaties, and shoed me away, like flicking away a fly at a picnic. Holding on as mightily as I could gained me nothing. When I flew backwards, away from Him, He looked at me and said one last thing, the only thing I remember distinctly, which is a shame because we spoke for what seemed like half an hour. Later, I struggled to remember everything He said, but His final injunction to me is all I could ever recall. I felt like I went to the well, but returned with only a spoonful of knowledge. While we spoke, He said many things that I remember being amazed and surprised at, but I was never able to remember what they were. His final words to me were, **"It is important that you help other people, without any expectation of reward."**

I took this final injunction to heart. It has been my Polaris, my guide star. Knowing that God will see my every deed and every thought again one day has kept me very circumspect, but no one can judge themselves, as I learned. I believe God's final words apply to everyone equally. Before my experience, I didn't have faith that

God existed. I tried to work up a religious fire when I was young, but blind faith proved an impossibility for me. Now that I have proof of God, all my doubts and suspicions have vanished. I know that God exists, that there is life after death, and that we must each face His judgment. How I live will determine if I pass or fail that judgment again. My experience was very telling in several respects. It showed me that despite my heathen ways, redemption is attainable through kindness to others. We can only take to heaven what we give away while we are here This is good news for everyone. The idea of helping others seems very New Testament. God requires no particular belief to earn His acceptance. If we can gain entry into heaven simply by being a good giving person, this would put all "men of the cloth" out of work. I told a long time student of Christianity about my experience. He offered to "interpret" my experience for me. I politely refused. My experience seemed straight forward and plain enough. It needed no "interpretation" or "spin". His offer seemed presumptuous and arrogant. My experience with God showed me heaven is open to all, 24 hours a day. Come as you are. No waiting. Accept no substitutes.

This is important because it shows that attitudes, beliefs, value systems and oaths mean absolutely nothing in the eyes of God. God doesn't play favorites. Rituals,

Robes and rugs will not earn your salvation. Save your money, save your time, and save your soul. Help people. Why God chose to enlighten me is a mystery. Surprisingly, I didn't suddenly get religion after my experience, but I did change my life. My subsequent volunteerism and helping those less able sprang from it. God's final words seem very much like the golden rule. If the path to heaven is this simple, why do we complicate it?

CHAPTER 8

A BRILLIANT IDEA

One evening the recovery team psychiatrist, Dr. Beth Johnson, came into my room to talk with me and see how I was getting on. After she sat down, she said, "I understand you're an author." "Yes, one of my books was published last year." I replied, still flushed with pride. "I saw your reviews. They're really very good. Have you thought of writing about your stroke and your experiences here?" she asked. "Well, sure," I admitted. "I've thought about it, but I don't know what I could bring to the party that would be new. All this business is new to me of course, but other people must have written about stroke and recovery. There must be several books on the market already." I said. "That's true," Dr. Johnson replied. "But, I see stroke patient's families every day who've just had a family member suffer a stroke or other traumatic brain injury and come here for rehabilitation. Those poor families are lost, and have no understanding of what their loved one is experiencing or how to help them. They're stressed out, and have lots of questions but no answers, so they turn to me for help. I do what I can, but if you wrote a book to help the families of survivors, sort of an insider's view of everything families should know, you could help a lot of people." Dr. Johnson said with conviction. She'd obviously thought about the idea a great deal. A book written to help survivor's families was something I hadn't considered. The more I thought about it, the better I liked it. It would be a way of obeying God's final injunction, and something more tangible than my volunteerism. There should have been a clap of thunder right then because the idea seemed too perfect, like an opportunity sent by God. Because of my lability, I started crying, unable to control the flood of emotions I was feeling. I was so happy and thrilled at the opportunity to help people that I couldn't contain my joy. The idea seemed absolutely perfect. Jeanine Reder, a talented speech pathologist on the recovery team stopped by just after Dr. Johnson left. I must have looked pretty strange, awash in tears and bawling like a sick calf. I tried to explain myself, but it was difficult between sobs. I felt like an idiot, but what could I do? I liked Jeanine and trusted her, so I just let it rip. I'm glad she was there, because I felt I had to tell someone about Dr. Johnson's brilliant idea and Jeanine was kind enough to listen. Each day I feel blessed because of this wonderful opportunity. So you see, when

I say my stroke was the best thing that ever happened to me, I truly mean it. I've been given a rare opportunity to help those who need it. You and others can judge whether I've successfully answered my charge.

CHAPTER 9

TAKING OWNERSHIP OF RECOVERY

After my miraculous escape from Hell, I took ownership of my recovery and became totally committed, not simply involved. It's like the old joke about the pig and the chicken who decide to make breakfast. The pig was committed and died supplying the bacon, while the chicken was only involved and laid a couple eggs. When I realized I was the biggest stakeholder in my therapy, I became one hundred percent committed to my recovery. To say I was an interested party is grievous understatement. Because my future would be defined by the outcome of my therapies, I took total ownership and responsibility for my recovery. I was surprised to learn some stroke patients don't understand why they are in hospital or why they're in therapy. They just don't get it. Some don't think they need therapy. Can you imagine the difficulty making a meaningful recovery for those people? This level of denial is terribly counterproductive and doesn't bode well for the patient's future prospects.

I had a brain injured friend in hospital who didn't think he belonged there. One day he told me he fell asleep and forgot his memory. His statement surprised me and made me laugh. I don't know if he ever remembered his memory. He told me often his brain was bad. This peculiar comment tickled me, too. I imagined him scolding his bad brain. Bad brain! Bad! Go to your room! You've been very bad today! My friend felt he was wrongly accused of having brain damage because he had a closed head injury. He didn't have a cool scar like mine. I wasn't sure if he belonged there or not, but I knew I did. I'm very thankful I was.

It is vital the survivor understand what has happened to them and understand why they need therapy. A survivor must be enlisted to work on his own behalf and must be a willing accomplice in their own rehabilitation. Rehabilitation is hard work. It can be agonizing, frustrating, and depressing. It is not fun. Recovery can be very slow, and every inch is hard won ground. When the survivor finally regains abilities to pre-injury levels, it's inspiring to see the transition from disabled to enabled. It takes courage and commitment to rehabilitate someone and give them wings.

Every stroke survivor and brain injury is unique, as is every recovery. One year after my stroke I still have some impairment. In my stroke support group I met a woman who is still struggling for recovery five years after her injury, though she has made remarkable progress. I also met a man who continues to fight for full recovery ten years after his injury. He's dejected because his recovery seems to have stopped. I'm sharing some recovery secrets with him I was lucky enough to learn. In the chapter titled Wishful Thinking I explain my unorthodox method of recovery. It worked well for me. He said he'd try it, but who knows? The psychological aspects of recovery are a trial, but I think he'll make it. So will you.

I've avoided talking about the hallucinations I experienced because talking about hallucinations is sorta like talking about dreams. "Who cares?" But, because I had hallucinations, perhaps others will experience them too, so I'll share my Foo Dog experience with you. Until I saw them and researched them, I didn't know what they were. Foo Dogs are mythological Chinese guard dogs. Statues of Foo Dogs are often seen outside the entrance of Chinese restaurants, Chinese businesses, and Chinese homes. I first saw them in Cholon, the Chinese district of Saigon, during the war but I didn't know what they represented. I think they were often painted red and looked like stylized lions, because of their exaggerated features and ferocious stance. Foo Dogs are considered good luck by the Chinese and are meant to frighten evil spirits from passing, just as gargoyles are used in Europe.

Foo Dogs are hideously ugly, with two tongues, fearsome teeth, piecing vigilant eyes, and a snarling threatening expression. They look like something straight out of hell.

As I was leaving the hospital in Bismarck before going to the Minneapolis VA Medical Center, I saw a little Foo Dog shoot across the floor like a rat and disappear into a wall. It was small, about eight inches tall, and moved fast, like it was on skates. I saw it three or four times in half an hour as I was leaving. I didn't tell anyone because I was afraid it would delay my discharge from the hospital and prevent my transfer to the VA Medical Center. I didn't see the little suckers after the transfer, so I wasn't particularly concerned. After my vision was miraculously restored, I began seeing lots of large Foo Dogs sitting on window sills, sitting on wall lockers and sitting on cabinets in the corridors around the hospital. A corridor might have ten or fifteen of them along either side. These were now big, perhaps five feet tall, and hideously ugly. I didn't see them move like the little ones had. They just watched me as I walked past them on my way to and from my various therapies. They were sorta transparent gray, and I could see through them. The way their eyes followed me was creepy, even though I knew they were just hallucinations. After almost a week of seeing big Foo Dogs, I went to Doctor Weber and told her I was hallucinating. That day she prescribed anti-seizure medication because she suspected my brain was having seizures. Shortly after I began taking the medication, the Foo Dogs disappeared. I wasn't troubled by Foo Dogs again. If you're having hallucinations, tell your doctor. I don't know how common hallucinations are for stroke survivors, but because the brain is insulted by stroke, it makes sense that hallucinations can occur. Mine were distracting and scary. I'm glad I spoke with Dr. Weber about them. Her diagnosis was spot on, and just what the doctor ordered.

CHAPTER 10

HOSPITAL ROUTINE

I worked hard in my therapies and wanted desperately to succeed. Each day the medical team made rounds through the wards and spoke with us individually to see how we were doing. Once a week, the Rehab team of doctors and therapists met to discuss individual patient progress. It was important that Dr. Weber have a thorough understanding of how each of us was progressing. Patients learn to compensate for their impairments. For my memory problems, Jeanine Reder gave me a day timer so I could write notes to myself, record appointments, meetings, and important dates. During the weekly team meetings I would be at the mercy of my therapists giving an accurate report of my efforts. Luckily my reports were accurate and testing played a big role in determining my progress. From these meetings I was given a list of goals the team expected me to meet before I would be considered ready for discharge. It was sort of like a parole from prison. "Inmate does not work and play well with others." The team goal was to only discharge patients capable of living and surviving in the real world. I was amazed at the close cooperation and communication among the various team members. Everyone was signing off the same sheet of paper, so there were never any mixed messages concerning what I needed to work on. I was always given a copy of my goals, and I worked on them assiduously so I could be discharged as quickly as possible. This staff synchronization was the result of Dr. Weber's skillful leadership. It was personally reassuring that the team worked so well together. I felt like I was in good hands with Dr. Weber's team. Mary Sullivan, my case manager, was Dr. Weber's priceless Major Domo. Mary worked hard to make certain things ran as they should. For instance, I was prescribed nicotine gum when I was trying to stop smoking, but it was rationed out by the nurses as if they were handing out their family jewels. This malarkey was irritating and silly. I had to beg just to get support to help me stop smoking. Mary Sullivan understood my frustration and went to bat for me. She got me relief pronto. I felt like chewing my leg off to shake my craving for nicotine. When my gum supply became regular, I stopped my escapes and played by the rules. Thank God for Mary's intervention. I was still dazed and confused. Having to pull pranks or beg for medication made each day a trial. With my nicotine addiction pacified with gum, I had no reason to go AWOL or jump the reservation.

Chapter 11

A Recognition Lesson

Stroke can create surprising impairments. My recovery was hindered somewhat because I'm hard-headed. I call it determined, but others have called me hard-headed and stubborn. I come by my stubbornness honestly enough; a deep vein of it runs in my family. From my family oral history comes this story of hard-headedness, stubbornness and determination. Many years ago, my grandfather, a poor Arkansas farmer, was gleaning a corn field, driving a balky mule pulling a wagon. Halfway across the harvested corn field, the mule stopped pulling and refused to move any further. Grandfather applied all the encouragement he could, popping the reins repeatedly until he was sweating from his exertions. Granddad shouted at Mr. Mule, cursed him, called him names, and then presented a litany of well reasoned arguments as to why the mule should resume his labors. I'm certain grandfather's eloquence, passion and reasoned opinion would have done any country lawyer proud, but Mr. Mule remained unconvinced. The insubordinate beast stood still as a lawn ornament despite granddad's entreaties, blandishments and threats, which only increased granddad's building fury. From experience, Grandpa knew the mule was particularly smart, and understood English language perfectly well. Granddad felt the mule was malingering just for spite. Soon this idea took root and festered in his mind until grandpa was hopping mad at the effrontery of the seditious beast. It was a test of wills with the ungrateful animal, which Granddad felt he should win. The mule was defying him just for pure meanness. Grandfather could be just as stubborn as Mr. Mule, and by jiggers, he'd prove it. That's when granddad had a brilliant idea. He decided to build a fire under the mule, and carefully erected a fine ziggurat beneath the mule using field detritus, desiccated corn stalks, withered corn cobs, dry shucks and likely looking weeds. When the structure was tall enough to match his fury, Granddad gleefully put a match to his creation, and rapidly climbed up onto the wagon seat, grabbed aholt of the reins and braced himself for the movement he knew would follow. When Mr. Mule felt the heat on his belly, he got the message pronto, made one energetic lunge forward, and then stopped again while he cooled. The lurch had positioned the wagon directly above the blaze, where it soon began to smolder and catch fire. Grandpa, his Vesuvian temper already running at full pressure, instantly understood the need for haste if the wagon was to be saved, and raged with renewed fury, as if he was battling Old Scratch himself. Suddenly, Grandpa snatched up an old rusty claw-hammer from the wagon box, leaped from the seat and jumped in front of Mr. Mule, where he shook the hammer in the mule's face, and screamed, "Move or die!" This was the ultimate test of Mr. Mule's linguistic abilities. The mule understood Granddad's lingo perfectly well, because he bolted away like Sea Biscuit out of the starting gate, and moved with purpose. He raced away with remarkable vigor leaving Granddad at the starting gate. Grandpa ran after the fleeing mule and the smoking wagon, shouting with every hop, and shaking his hammer at the contrary son of a gun. He knew if he didn't catch up quick, his only wagon might burn to the ground. At stressful times like this, Granddad got creative linguistically and invented new cuss words the world had never heard. This was the dawn of creation. Granddad was clever that way. He surely felt like Thomas Edison, on the cusp of inventive greatness. The one or two onlookers (my uncles) couldn't guess what the words meant, but the tone and tenor sounded awful bad. Panting heavily, Granddad finally reached the smoldering wagon after a fair chase, and wheezed to a stop beside it at the end of the field, where Mr. Mule stood exhausted, and blowing heavily from the strain of the chase. The poor thing was all done in. Granddad threw down his hammer, dropped to the ground, and began slinging dirt on the smoking and smoldering bits of undercarriage, like a badger in spring time. In the end, the wagon and the half bushel of feed corn it held, were saved. The Arkansas-Hairless racing mule eventually healed up, and his hair grew back in. Granddad used to laugh about Mr. Mule and boast that, if more speed was needed, all he had to do was to pick up a hammer in sight of the beast.

When I was told I'd have certain impairments because of my stroke, I'd argue and deny it. Telling me I won't be able to do simple stuff I learned as a child was ridiculous and made me mad. I often gave the news bearer some grief, too. This reaction to news of impairments is common among stroke survivors. When I was told I'd have certain impairments, my initial reaction was to lash out and give the therapist some gas. Often, I'd insult successive generations of the therapist's family and question their chromosome count. It's human nature to resent a steady flow of bad tidings and the people who keep bringing it. To expect otherwise is folly. Greeting more bad news with a cheery smile is simply not in me. Eventually, the abused and gun shy staff decided to let me discover my impairments in my own way. This was wise and much easier on everyone involved.

What follows is how I discovered an impairment by myself. It's an ugly tale, but true. One day following rounds, a woman came into my room dressed in a white smock like every doctor, nurse, therapist, clerk, cook and gardener. "Hi," she said cheerfully, "I'm doctor Torne-Perez, with a hyphen. How are you doing today?" she asked. "Oh, hi! I'm doing great," I replied, as she began checking the muscle tone in my arms and legs. "The nicotine gum is working out alright then?" she asked. "Yes, it's working fine," I confirmed. Dr. Perez spoke with a slight accent that interested me very much, because I couldn't quite place it, and I used to be pretty good at identifying accents. I wondered, *"Do I have a mystery to solve here?"*

"You're still using the 4 milligram dosage of nicotine gum then?" The doctor with a hyphen asked, still pinching and poking my muscles.

"Yes, that gum is a miracle. Any time I get the itch for a smoke, I just chew a piece of gum," I said proudly, like I'd invented the stuff. A tiny cartoon angel should have appeared on my shoulder and whispered in my ear, *"Hey! Don't let your alligator mouth overload you hummingbird hind parts!"*

"I'm so happy you've stopped smoking. You're doing very good too," she continued, patting my arm. "how would you feel if I lowered the dosage?" the doctor asked me, "I'd like to see you use a lower dosage. Would that be alright?"

"You're the doctor. If you think I should switch to low octane, I will, if you think I should," I offered graciously. "I never thought I could do this well, so I'm in your hands doctor!" "Great, I'll write new orders, and see how you do," she reassured. "Let me know if there's a problem. Doctor Weber is away for the weekend, so I'll get those new orders taken care of today. I don't think she will have a problem with them," Dr. Torne-Perez said with her pleasant accent. "Where are you from doctor? You have a nice accent, but I can't quite place it. It's very beautiful," I said. "Oh, thank you," I'm from Columbia and Panama." she said, and seemed mildly surprised that I would ask.

"Since Columbia used to own Panama, that makes sense," I said. I'd learned this tidbit while doing research for an earlier book. I figured I was one of two people in the country who were aware of this historic oddity. Author's note: Here's where all idiots on the boat jump overboard. *If I'd been smart, I 'd have tied the anchor around my neck and jumped in, too!* She was very nice and I secretly hoped to impress her with my boundless knowledge of her native land. The only people in my room I could talk with were a sick old man across from me and a pain in the butt Texan in the bed next to mine, who'd been admitted with terminal constipation. He quickly exhausted my knowledge of, or interest in, Country Western music. A nice guy, but jeeze, what a pain in the fanny. His bellarin' kept me awake at night. With an accent like his, I expected something more, profound thoughts maybe, or road wisdom. Give me something, anything! Because I watched the History Channel every hour of the day on the ancient steam powered television we shared, he said he was going to be too smart when he went home, and that threw me into a mental tailspin. How exactly can a Texan be too smart? Learn to cipher with his boots on? Read without moving his lips? That was a year and a half ago and I'm still bothered by it.

Okay, I was starved for conversation and diversion, so I started skylarking a little bit with the pretty lady doctor. I admit it. This woman was like a cool breeze blowing into the room. No harm, no foul.

"Actually I grew up in Columbia, but my mother is from Panama, so I've spent time there as well," she said, unimpressed, not rising to my jeopardy trivia. I wanted to chitchat, but I cleverly resisted the urge to talk about illegal drugs.

"Huh. I graduated from the School of the Americas in Chagres, Panama. Its very beautiful there, lots of wildlife. I loved the jungle and the wildlife," I said, throwing another scrap out, as if she didn't know Panama had lots of wildlife. This lady was attractive and fun to talk with. Her slight accent was killer! I loved it! *Intriguing yet captivating, I thought and imagined waggling my eyebrows like Senior Groucho. Just then, I had an odd thought and wondered, what would Pepe La Pew do to demonstrate his infatuation? He'd grab her hand, kiss her wrist, and then work his way up her arm, showering her right slam up to her armpit. Next, he'd give her other hand and arm more of the same.* Author's note: Beginners must be careful not to slobber and drool. *Then, Pepe would utter the most famous line ever spoken in Pidgin English, "Come, come weez me to zee Kazbah. We weel make beautiful muzik togezer."*

"Huh?" I asked, snapping out of my cartoon reverie. I don't usually take my cues from cartoon characters, but that little overripe French sleaze was such a romantic fool, he made me laugh. "Everything else is alright?" she asked. "Oh, I'm sorry, I didn't hear you. I guess I was daydreaming," I said lamely. Darn, strike two. "I tried to walk down to the vending room last night to get a soft drink, but the nurses on the desk wouldn't let me go without an escort. Do you think I could be allowed to leave the ward occasionally?" I asked innocently. "I'd like to move around a little bit."

"Absolutely! I'll write new orders for you when I change the notes for your gum. Let me know how the gum works out." she said, and fttt! She was gone. Wow! I liked her. *Huba huba!* The pounding in my ears was my heart. The doctor was very gentle and ladylike, with delicate, almost birdlike movements. She was refined, sophisticated, polished. She was an adult, and she wasn't mental. *She must be very bright to be a doctor*, I thought to myself. I'm pretty quick with the obvious stuff, huh? I daydreamed shamelessly of taking her home, like something I'd won at the county fair. "Hey Dad, look what I found! I like her!" That evening I walked down to the vending area and had my first Coke in nearly two months. It was disorienting, moving around in unfamiliar areas, but so refreshing! *Freedom! Yip Yip Yippie!! Montanans don't actually say this junk, but I've seen enough old movies to know I should. I think I fling my cap up right here for emphasis! "Thank you doctor Torne-Perez, wherever you are, thank you and good night!"* to paraphrase Jimmy Durante's old schtick.

The following day, Saturday, a woman I'd never seen, swept into my room and asked how I was doing. "I'm doing great!" "I got to leave the ward last night without an escort!" I gushed to her proudly. "Good! What did you do?" she asked. "One of the doctors changed my orders so I could move around a little bit," I said excitedly. "So I went down to the vending room and bought my first Coke in months. It was terrific! I'm thankful the doctor trusted me." "Yes, that was me," the woman said, in sotto voce without moving her lips, like a ventriloquist. I didn't know what she meant or if she was speaking to me, so I ignored her. "You know, trust is really important between doctor and patient, so I wanted the doctor to know she could rely on me, and that I can be trusted," I explained. "Yes, that was me," she said again, but I still didn't understand. *Why is she saying this stuff? Is she speaking to me?* I wondered again, still at a loss for an answer that made sense. I decided to ignore her once more, because I was flustered by the sotto voce ventriloquist business. If I'd had longer hair, it would have stood straight up about now, because I was freaked out. "I see by your orders you've started with the reduced nicotine gum. Is that working alright for you?" the new lady doctor asked. "So far, so good," I replied smiling, happy to be part of a conversation I understood. "I 'm excited about being able to leave the ward. The other doctor did me huge when she changed my orders." I crowed. "Yes, that was me," the lady doctor said again, without moving her lips! All my mental alarms were going off because I knew something wasn't right. My sense of disorientation and dislocation was absolute. Just then, the lady doctor leaned forward and looked at me closely, like I was a rare hothouse retard. Then, the germ of an idea seeped into my brain, just a possibility at first, and then a suspicion. As it matured, the realization was almost physically painful. *The woman*

*before me is the same woman I spoke with yesterday, the doctor
from Columbia and Panama, Dr. Torne-Perez!* She didn't look
the same! She looked totally different! Did she change
her hair? Shave her beard? What the hell is going on?
How could I not recognize her? Where is her beautiful
accent? Is this a trick? People shouldn't be allowed to
impersonate themselves by not looking like them! This
is creepy! I would swear I've never seen this woman in
my life, but reluctantly I guessed maybe I had. I am such
an idiot, talking to her and about her at the same time, in
some sort of sick first person third person double back-
flip. Toss in a little past tense and present tense like I
did and you got a helluva mess! Jeeze, I spoke to her as
though she wasn't a party to our conversation the day
before! I looked more closely at her, as the incredible truth
sunk into my single functioning brain cell. *Oh God, I am
an idiot!* I thought to myself, over and over, as I reached
desperately for a painless face-saving escape. *How can I
possibly play this off?* Nothing floated up, no great idea.
My brain simply stopped. Then the image of Yosemite
Sam with smoke rolling out of his pants floated up, and
Sam suddenly shouts "My biscuits are burnin'!", when he
realizes his pants are on fire. Right then, I knew exactly
how Sam felt. This wasn't a cartoon, but I did the only
thing I could. I decided to ignore the lady once more, and
brass it out, as if I was normal, and hope she wouldn't

notice. I was so embarrassed, I wished I could have simply disappeared. *"I hope she doesn't report this,"* I thought to myself. I could just imagine what her report would say. *"Patient is delusional, unaware of his surroundings, and a complete idiot!"* In North Carolina, some bubba would say of me, "Nope, this boy just ain't right. He ain't got the brains God gave a gopher!" It's more than a year since my stroke. I still don't recognize people I've met before. I'll gladly meet someone for the second time and then hustle through the introductions hoping they won't notice. If they do, I feign total surprise. "Well, good to meet you again then!" I reply heartily, hoping they'll think my eyes are playing tricks on them. My solution isn't perfect, but it's better than doing nothing, which amounts to an admission of retardation. I suspect some people I've met have this conversation with their wife, "Remember that retard I met for the first time twice last week?" I met him for the first time again last night. I wish I knew what's going on." *Me too. I'm developing a recognition complex, with a twitch to match.*

CHAPTER 12
COMMON REHABILITATION THERAPIES

The goal of rehabilitation therapies is survivor independence. Stroke is devastating psychologically, mentally and physically. A comprehensive regime of therapy should address all three of these areas. When someone suffers a traumatic brain injury they must relearn just about everything. Having to relearn simple tasks they learned as a child is demoralizing. The survivor's understanding and acceptance of their condition comes through testing and therapy as they struggle with even simple tasks they've done all their lives. When the survivor discovers the depth and scope of their impairments, their self-image and confidence will be shaken.

This self-discovery process is absolutely necessary so the survivor can understand their true capabilities. If a therapist had told me I wouldn't be able to do even simple tasks I'd done since childhood, I wouldn't have believed them. In fact, I probably would have gotten angry with them for low-balling me and treating me like a child.

No survivor wants to believe they are so crippled, so impaired, so dependent. Part and parcel of therapy is testing to determine what capabilities have been lost and what capabilities remain. Testing clearly demonstrates to the survivor their limitations. As the survivor improves and becomes more able through therapy, testing confirms any improvement, and treatment decisions can be made based on facts, not feelings.

What follows are descriptions of standard therapies used by most institutions with Stroke rehabilitation programs, except Tai Chi. This is not presently a standard therapy, but I feel it should be. Tai Chi is slowly gaining acceptance as a viable physical therapy for stroke rehabilitation.

Each of the therapies that follow was part of my daily rehabilitation routine while I was a patient at the Minneapolis VA Medical Center. Each therapy session was half an hour or one hour long. This means that I had physical therapy every weekday while I was in hospital. The same is true of the other therapies. I've taken the long way around the barn to explain that every rehabilitation patient needs a great deal of training. Rehabilitating someone after a stroke is a major undertaking. Lots of work and time are needed. Many survivors lose track of time and have no sense of continuity, or flow, or connectedness of days or dates or months. This is tough to explain because time seems so basic to everyone. Not to stroke survivors. This is why many of my therapists would begin each session with simple questions about time. "What day is this? What is the date? What season is this? Tell me the days of the week backwards from today. What month is this? Tell me the months in the year backwards from this month." Not all these simple questions involve time, but most do. "Count from one hundred backwards. Tell me all the letters of the alphabet backwards. Using these simple tests the therapist can get an understanding of how the patient is functioning cognitively. I believe many therapies can be done at home if the caregiver is a well informed and skilled observer. There are computer programs available that may help with some therapies. There are other programs that help with testing along the way. Therapy professionals and the resources in this book can help you find answer to these two questions, "Can I help my loved one with therapy at home? Must I hire a professional therapist?" The efficacy of any therapy is determined by the results, and the time and effort it took to get a satisfactory result. As a nonprofessional therapist, you really don't know what the outcome of your efforts will be. Will home therapy be a huge waste of everyone's time? Who knows? Who can say? Call the organizations I've listed in the Help for Survivors and Families chapter using their free eight hundred numbers and put your questions to them. They can give you specific answers.

It is important to remember the survivor may have to relearn many things. As they relearn forgotten skills, their confidence will grow and they will slowly become more independent. Be patient with your survivor. Praise their hard work, and reward their efforts.

TAI CHI

I was asked to evaluate Tai Chi (pronounced "ty chee") while I was in hospital to see if it would be appropriate for stroke patients. I think Tai Chi would be wonderful. It would help with body awareness, which many survivors have lost. Tai Chi would help develop balance, something many survivors struggle with. Tai Chi would develop flexibility and strengthen muscles. Tai Chi places emphasis on visualization and can use guided imagery. There are many Tai Chi video tapes available, but you'll need to be selective about which you choose. I think it is important that a good video discuss Chi energy. This same energy is called Ki (pronounced "key") by the Japanese and is the basis of Aikido, a true martial art but very soft because it has no striking or kicking. Tai Chi has a limited number of "positions" or movements, which can be learned relatively fast. They have poetic sounding names like "Wind in the Willows," "Combing the Horses Mane" and "Waves Crashing on Rocks." Tai Chi is similar to a Martial Art but, because it has no impact, no throws, and no contact of any kind, it is not and should not be considered a Martial Art. Tai Chi is almost like ballet, or "statues," and anyone should be able to learn it. This ancient Chinese exercise has a rich history and millions of people, many of whom are well into old age, practice it daily. With no strikes, kicks, throws, holds or grappling, someone may get their feelings hurt if you make a face at them, but that's about all. For stroke survivors, Tai Chi brings a lot to the party. I recommend it unequivocally. I suspect Tai Chi could be the only physical therapy needed for the rehabilitation of stroke survivors.

PHYSICAL THERAPY

I had a stroke on the right hemisphere of my brain. My impairments are very different from a survivor who had an injury on their left hemisphere. It's important to remember a stroke survivor continues to heal and improve for approximately one year after their injury. While I was in hospital, I began daily physical therapy where my abilities were assessed and tested. My ability to take and follow directions was tested, as well as my ability to climb stairs, balance, visually scan, lift weights, and orient myself. My speed was a big issue because I was very slow after the stroke. I walked and moved slowly. Another part of physical therapy was direction finding. My therapist and I took long walks and I practiced finding my way around the grounds and area, including nearby neighborhoods.

All this may sound easy, but it wasn't. My therapist grew up in the city and knew nothing of the trees and plants we passed on our walks, so I identified the different trees and plants if I knew them. This gave me a sense of familiarity and was very relaxing. My therapist vapor-locked when we passed under a mulberry tree and I reached up and started snacking on the delicious, unusually sweet, ripe berries. She refused to try one. I'd been taught outdoor skills all my life. I suppose my therapist had no one to teach her basic outdoor survival skills. I identified different plants first used by native Americans for their medicinal value, and explained the uses of each as I knew them. Things like Elm, maple, and spruce, long needle pine, vervain, summack, chokecherry, milkweed, yarrow, burrdock, hemlock, cattail and spearmint were all within our walk. My impatient therapist was very demanding, like an Army drill instructor with bad hemorrhoids. She had the itch to move on, and saw no value in nature or its uses. The homily was right, you really can't make 'em drink after you've led them to water. She seemed determined to work me to a frazzle, which she did, much to her quiet delight. She did me good despite my "laxadaisical" attitude. She just didn't appreciate my Camp Counselor routine. She wanted me to work, not forage for snacks. Direction finding is a common problem for some stroke survivors. We get lost and confused easily, making getting around very troublesome. The visual cues everyone takes for granted when they make their way around are overlooked and less obvious for us. We simply don't notice or remember them, so finding our way around is a big problem. If we walk too fast and don't have time to study all the landmarks then we can't remember them. If things are moving too fast, I can't find my way again because "I'm slow, you silly cow!"

Many survivors lose the use of their limbs because they've lost motor control in their brain. A new therapy called BATRAC[16], which stands for Bilateral Repetitive Rhythmic Training Intervention is showing very positive results. Survivors who had this training actually had increased brain activity as shown by magnetic resonance imaging (MRI) on both the injured and the uninjured side of the brain. This is good news because it suggests that lost control can be gained through proper therapeutic stimulation. I lost full control of my left leg and left arm to my stroke but I forced myself to keep using them as well as I was able. I eventually regained their full use because I would not accept their loss without a fight. It was a close thing though. When I was first put in hospital, I was put in a wheelchair.

I refused to cede my limbs to the stroke, so I worked hard to regain their full use. Certainly I was clumsy and spastic looking, but now you'd never know I ever had a problem. I was determined to minimize the debilitating effects of the stroke as well as I could. Much impairment I was able to overcome, or I learned compensations to mitigate their impact on my life as much as possible. I still have a left field cut, but with extra scanning I have reduced its impact on the quality of my life. I hope one day to eliminate the field cut entirely.

So far, my vision has improved, but I still have work to do. I continue to work for total recovery. I have no idea if I'll be successful, but what should I do? Give up? There is absolutely no way I'll stop working to restore my abilities. I want my life back! I can think of no better way to spend my time than working toward this goal. I also exercise twice a day to restore my thinking to pre-stroke levels. My cognitive abilities have improved tremendously. I have more work to do though, so I continue my exercises and will until I can no longer do them.

I explain my personal recovery methodologies in the chapter titled Wishful Thinking, if you're interested in "self-help".

OCCUPATIONAL THERAPY

This therapy involves "life skills" such as cooking, food preparation, shopping, driver's testing, direction finding, making correct change, dressing properly, personal care, using the telephone, the yellow pages, and other general life skills. These therapists also did lots of testing so, as the patient improves, test results can be compared and improvements noted. Numerous outings helped remind us of the real world out there.

I had a nice Mexican friend in this therapy named Valensuela. A great guy, but our therapist insisted on calling him Mr. Venezuela. That she would call my friend by the name of a country used to crack us up, but my friend wasn't upset in the least. The therapist just didn't get it. Valensuela, Venezuela, what difference does it make? None to my friend. He was very generous and overlooked her blunders graciously.

This same therapist took a group of us to the market so we could do the therapist's grocery shopping. The tight budget made us work hard to stretch each dollar. "If corn on the cob is twenty three cents a pound, how much will it cost if I get just three ears?" "Huh?" This sounded suspiciously like "Who's on First." I couldn't solve for x in my head, so I gave up and risked a bad report. With a calculator, it wouldn't have been a problem. Everyone got disgusted and walked outside, where we waited to return to the safety and sanity of the hospital. I felt so obvious standing there, like a fish out of water. I felt like all of us were a dead give-away with our wander alarms and hospital code bracelets. My fresh craniotomy scar marked me plainly as a head case. I felt like I was in the fishing-boat scene from "One Flew Over the Cuckoos Nest." I felt so obvious, and I hated it. I felt I stuck out like a sore thumb, way different from normal. It was a terrible feeling. I couldn't wait until we left and the trial ended. I remember going through the checkout line and chipping in money for the therapist because she had no more. I gave her everything I had just to make the ordeal end quickly. The newness of going out shopping after months in hospital felt very weird and very foreign. It sorta gave me the creeps. All the products were visually confusing when I tried to find specific items like cold medicine or toothpaste. None of this should have been a problem, but it took extra time for me to scan because of my left field cut and terrible vision.

Here in North Dakota, pronunciation is sometimes problematic. All the weather girls on radio and television have trouble pronouncing the word meteorologist. I don't know if their tongues stumble over their bridge work or what, but most of them add a sudden pause, and say "meaty urologist." When I think what a meaty urologist might be it gives me the shudders. Folks here have no accent, so I found this linguistic quirk interesting.

SPEECH THERAPY

While still a patient at the Veterans Affairs Medical Center in Minneapolis, I issued a call for papers to the staff because I wanted input from doctors, therapists and nurses for this book before I'd written anything. As a patient, all I knew of the various therapies was what I'd experienced or what I found in my research. Jeanine Reder, my wonderful speech therapist, submitted the following for my use here, and I appreciate her generous assistance.

Speech therapists, otherwise known as Speech-Language Pathologists, do much more than the title suggests. Speech therapists do indeed help people who have speech or communication difficulties after a stroke, but they also may help people with swallowing and/or cognitive impairments suffered as a result of a stroke. Frequently after a stroke, people may have trouble eating and/or swallowing. This is due to the fact that many of the same muscles which control speech also control eating and/or swallowing. This particular type of disorder is called <u>dysphagia</u>. This can be dangerous if the survivor is getting food or liquid into their airway (<u>aspiration</u>). If food or liquid finds its way to the lungs, a person may develop an <u>aspiration pneumonia</u>. Speech therapists often evaluate and treat people after a stroke to ensure they can swallow safely. If not, they may recommend modifying the texture of the diet to make it safer. Speech therapists also help treat many other types of impairments suffered as a result of a stroke. The type of impairments vary depending on which side or <u>hemisphere</u> of the brain was affected by the stroke, as well as which particular area of the brain was damaged. For instance, people who have left-hemisphere strokes can have quite different impairments from someone who has suffered a right-hemisphere stroke. Common impairments after a left-hemisphere include difficulty speaking or finding words, and/or trouble understanding language. This type of impairment is called <u>asphasia</u>. This language impairment can affect all areas of language. Asphasia can impair not only speaking, and listening, but also reading and writing. Often times if a person has asphasia they may also have what is called an <u>apraxia of speech</u>. Apraxia of speech is a motor-programming problem. The muscles work, but the muscles which control speech movements goes awry. Another type of speech disorder which can occur in either a left or right-hemisphere stroke is called <u>dysarthria.</u> Dysarthria is a weakness or paralysis in the muscles which control speech. There are several different types of dysarthrias, each dependent upon the part of the brain affected by the stroke. A typical example of dysarthria is slurred speech after a stroke.

Impairments after a right-hemisphere stroke can vary from person to person in type and severity, just like left-hemisphere stroke. Some common impairments seen after a right-hemisphere stroke include difficulty paying attention to the right side of the body or environment on the right. This is called neglect. These people may often bump into things on their right because of their diminished awareness/attention to that side. Visual field deficits are also commonly seen after a right-hemisphere stroke. Other types of impairments seen in this type of stroke include difficulty interpreting emotions from facial expression and/or speech prosody. The stroke survivor may lack prosody or melody in their speech. They may have a flat, monotonous quality to their speech. They also may have difficulty interpreting humor. They may have difficulty understanding implied meanings in conversations and metaphors. For example, the proverb "Don't count your chickens before they hatch." may literally mean "Okay, I had better wait until those chickens hatch before I count them." A person who has suffered a right-hemisphere stroke may also have difficulties with the social aspects of communication, or pragmatics. Eye contact may be poor and they may fail to allow the person to take a turn in conversation. Their speech may become rambling or off topic at times. The stroke can also affect a person's awareness of these impairments and they may lack insight and/or be in denial of any difficulties they are experiencing.

Impairments which are common in both left and

right-hemisphere strokes include attention impairments, memory disturbances, problem solving, planning/ organization and reasoning impairments. All of the above-mentioned impairments may vary from person to person in type and severity depending upon the type, location and severity of the stroke the person has suffered. Along with other members of the stroke rehabilitation team, the speech therapist may assist in evaluation and treating the patient suffering from many of their impairments. Together with time, hard work and therapy, most patients can achieve some improvement in their impairments. Of course, there are no guarantees, as no stroke is the same.

Submitted on 5/17/05 by: Jeanine M. Reder, M.S., CCC-SLP, Speech-Language Pathologist

REFERENCES

Brookshire, RH. *Introduction to Neurogenic Communication Disorders*, 5th Edition, St. Louis, 1997, Mosby.

Love, RJ, Webb, WG. *Neurology for the Speech Language Pathologist*, 3rd Edition, Newton, MA, 1996, Butterworth-Heinemann.

RECREATION THERAPY

Laura Barrett was my wonderful recreation therapist. It was her job to get long term patients like myself out of the dull hospital routine and involved doing things that interested us. Each time the stroke survivor moves to a different environment from the hospital, it's like doing it for the first time in the patient's life. Laura got me working on the internet and doing basic research for this book. In addition, she and I went to the history museum in St. Paul and visited the Mall of America where we had a decent meal, which was my first in more than a month. Laura had me practice my direction finding skills as well. She was also responsible for getting patients involved in such therapeutic activities as pizza parties, fishing, and going to films and other agreeable diversions. When you've had a stroke and spent months in hospital, each experience offers new challenges and is a learning experience as patients adapt and readjust to the real world. Laura was terrific at this and at getting patients involved in life. This was not all fun and games though. Each activity had its own challenges and difficulties the patient must overcome. It was in Laura's therapy that I got the chance to crow about art and design. Talking with a pretty woman always makes me feel better.

CHAPTER 13

CREATING A SAFE HARBOR

Here are some accommodations you may wish to make so the home is a more safe and a more healing environment for the stroke survivor:

SOFT MUSIC is healing and restorative. My brain felt very frazzled when I returned home. I felt relief just listening to soft music. Loud rock n' roll music was like a hacksaw in my brain.

ESTABLISH A FIXED ROUTINE for meal times, shopping, laundry and other interactions. This is very comforting to the survivor after they've learned the routine and brings certainty to an uncertain world. Any messages or information given to a survivor should be kept short or written down for a shorter attention span and poor memory.

HANDRAILS on stoops and stairs help because many survivors have balance and vision problems, making falls a real possibility. We often have physical weakness and railings are inexpensive insurance. Another head injury could prove disastrous. I've fallen four times down stairs or off stoops since returning home. Handrails saved me once, and railings would have saved me at other times. A trip down the stairs is not fun.

Night Lights help when we have to use the washroom during the night. They help prevent disorientation in the dark when we can't figure out where we are. It might also be helpful to **remove all throw rugs** to prevent tripping.

A Big Mirror in the bedroom is also helpful, because we have problems getting our clothes on and buttoned properly. A mirror allows us to "check our gig line" before we leave our area. No one enjoys walking around dressed like a retard. It looks bad.

A Big Wall Calendar is helpful because we often lose time sense. Make certain it's big enough to note appointments, birthdays, and such, so we don't miss a special day.

All this special accommodating may be irksome, but it makes life safer and less stressful. Independence is the goal. Being dependent on others is not fun. My biggest problem is my lack of mobility. I've always been independent. Now I have to mooch rides, use public transportation, or walk. Other helpful things include a **digital clock**, a **radio**, and a **rocking chair**.

A DIARY OR JOURNAL can be helpful because the survivor continues to change after their injury and they gradually recover. It's helpful for them to be able to see how they were at various stages of their recovery and just how much they've improved. I began keeping a journal while I was in hospital. I didn't know what to write and I didn't have any idea what would be important later, but I'm very glad I did because my journal became the basis for this book. As the survivor improves, it's easy to forget all their difficulties, trials, and the small victories that gave them hope for the future For some reason survivors will often share their diary with me. I suppose because I'm a writer and a survivor, they feel I would be interested. I am. In a small way, someone reading about their struggle validates their experience. When reading someone's diary I'm reading about their tragedy and their triumph, how they overcame their shocking reality and found courage to keep going. Some of their stories are absolutely Homeric, in terms of valor, and an unwillingness to quit when everything and everyone tells them they should. One woman gave me the diary she kept during her five year stroke recovery. The more I read the more proud I am of her for her marvelous recovery. Every survivor should keep a diary or journal of their voyage. They're inspiring for others and very cathartic for the writer.

A KITCHEN TIMER is helpful if the survivor is going to cook. I spoke with a survivor who uses a timer like this and she said it was very helpful. Because we have memory and attention problems, the expense is low cost safety. If I'm doing something, like cooking, I know I may forget my cooking and sit down to watch TV. This lady always sets her timer before she walks away from her stove. When the bell rings, she checks to see what she has going on the stove. This is a good plan, but takes discipline to work.

If I've heard "SHOWER CHAIR" once I've heard it a thousand times, because it's the most obvious accommodation. The survivor must bathe themselves and a shower chair is helpful to prevent falls.

A CALCULATOR WITH LARGE KEYS AND DISPLAY is also very helpful. Some survivors are like me and have difficulty with numbers. I have someone to help me with my banking and help me keep my checking account balanced. Because of my organization problems and my difficulty with numbers, a calculator helps.

A LARGE KEY TELEPHONE is helpful. Even dialing a telephone is confusing to me. It seems "alien" for some reason. The keypad gives me a very creepy feeling, like it belongs in a different world somehow. I can't explain it, I'm afraid, but just knowing I have to make a phone call makes me nervous. The calling card process gives me fits too, because so many numbers must be entered. The numbers on the card are tiny and hard to see. All the dialing makes my skin crawl. I get lost somehow dialing all those blasted numbers and lose track of where I am and what number I just entered. I've tried and failed repeatedly for hours sometimes. Not a fun process, and one of many reminders that I'm impaired.

If you take a stroke survivor out to dinner or some other place, quietly escort them slowly to the washroom and escort them back to their seat. Show them where you came into the building. I have horrible trouble becoming oriented and finding my way around in new surroundings. All the noise and movement of other people is very distracting, so help us out if you wouldn't mind.

KEEP THE NOISE DOWN in the home. Kids running through screaming are very nerve-racking, as is loud music. Soft soothing music will help the survivor relax and heal. This needn't last forever. After a few months of adjustment, we can handle most things just fine. We just need time to let our brain cool down.

MAKE SURE THE SURVIVOR GETS OUTSIDE. We all need exercise to maintain our health. If the survivor forgets this, remind them and take them for a walk or something.

I walk between 1 and 2 miles almost daily. See that your survivor exercises frequently. Their health is all they have. Have everyone's blood pressure checked frequently, including yours. Good mental health can be improved with lots of human socialization and interaction.

HELP THE SURVIVOR JOIN A STROKE SUPPORT GROUP. You can find one by calling your nearest hospital. The patient will meet others who've had similar experiences and will share what they've learned. These groups are extremely helpful and can suggest compensations they've learned for different impairments. This is where the patient learns how to make life tolerable. I can't say enough good things about support groups. They're wonderful. Having a positive attitude in group is critical. Each group will have its own personality. Some are upbeat but others can be depressing. The tone of the group is set by the group leader. It is their job to keep the group focused and not allow the group to dissemble into a whiners club. If you fall into a group of whiners, you can find a different group or you can change the focus of the group by enlisting the help of the group leader and working to get the group back on track. People sometimes fall into a rut and don't realize it. A stroke survivor has lost their entire world. They're stuck with the wreckage and must make the best of it. Psychologically adjusting to their handicapped status is difficult and stressful. We cannot think of everything and must rely on others. It's a rare person who can put themselves into the shoes of another successfully. I've never seen it done without a lot of stress, hurt feelings and strain on all concerned. Together, a working accommodation must be found between all parties. This is hard work. I'm forced to rely on others who have lives of their own to live. My dependence on them and lack of mobility are very troubling to me. If I'm out of toilet paper, toothpaste, laundry detergent and denture cleaner, I need to go to the store now! How about a lift?

Sometimes I make bad decisions. My clothes dryer played out today, so I had a couple loads of wash to dry. Hanging everything around my home screamed yard sale. It takes too long for everything to dry "naturally". Then, I remembered John Candy in the film "Uncle Buck" used a microwave to dry his clothes. Great idea! So, one evening, my microwave became my clothes dryer. No one likes damp undies. On my fifth or sixth load, I got impatient and turned up the power. After setting two pairs of drawers on fire, I hung everything around my place to dry. I didn't think it possible for damp cotton to burst into flames. I was amazed. The term "Chinese fire-drill" springs to mind.

If you take a survivor to market so they can shop, don't crowd them or rush them. Handicapped people are slow. We need more time because we're handicapped! If you're impatient or have ants in your pants, go sit someplace. You shouldn't have come along! Many survivors I've spoken with feel pressured when shopping. This is maddening and a miserable experience for us. Too often I get home with the wrong stuff, or missing things I wanted to pick up. Pressuring the handicapped with snide comments and feigned martyrdom and exasperation is childish, so grow up.

CHAPTER 14

SURVIVOR PSYCHOLOGY

Following a stroke, emotions can be difficult for the survivor to control because the stroke physiologically causes problems with crying and laughter. I had difficulty with lability, also called reflex crying, and I would cry suddenly with no warning of onset. Sudden laughing for no apparent reason, laughing longer than appropriate and laughing at inappropriate times can sometimes be a problem too. These emotional responses may subside in time or they may not. It is my feeling that lability and laughter usually subsides, but this could take years.

Stroke can cause clinical depression, feelings of sadness, hopelessness, helplessness, bitterness, anger, frustration, or anxiety may occur. The survivor's return home can be stressful for all concerned. The survivor has just passed through one of the most traumatic experiences they will ever face. They are often flooded with emotions, feelings of insecurity, and doubt. They've been shaken, and stressed beyond comprehension. The survivor can be uncertain about their adjustment from the safe, cloistered confines of the hospital, where the routine is well known and familiar. When moving to a different environment, even the home, there are many unknowns. Will the survivor be able to function? Will they be too much of a burden on the family? Will they need help? If so, how much, and how will they know? I couldn't wait to "graduate" from rehabilitation and return home, but I was filled with endless questions and uncertainties about my future. The longer the survivor has been away from home, the more difficult the return can be. I felt like a returning POW being repatriated at war's end. I've told you about the strangeness of a small market and how eerie it felt outside the hospital environment. Just being out of the familiar was very unsettling. My return home felt the same. Home felt very strange. It took months for the strangeness to dissipate and the comfort and security I'd previously known to return.

Adjusting to people and personal interactions took a considerable amount of time until everyone felt comfortable. I learned everyone must remain open and flexible while the feeling out process and adjustment period of exploring capabilities and limitations is under way. Feelings may get bruised, and wrongful assumptions may be made, but this period of adjustment is necessary until routines can be established, limitations determined, and boundaries are defined for everyone. Until this happens, daily life can be a little bumpy emotionally. Once everyone's routines, abilities and expectations are known, everyone can relax and stop trying so hard.

Survivors may be manipulative when working for personal goals. They are often transparent and obvious. Everyone likes to get their own way. Just because the survivor has had a difficult time doesn't mean they should get a free pass through life. You don't have to accept rudeness, antisocial behavior, or verbal or physical abuse from a survivor. Personality changes due to stroke can be shocking. If this becomes an issue, call the listings in the Resources for Survivors and Families chapter and get help.

I must repeat my warning about the high incidence of suicide among stroke survivors after they return home. Pay particular attention for signs of depression such as moodiness, irritability, muted happiness, underlying sadness, lack of spontaneous interaction, social withdrawal, changes in eating habits, isolation or seclusion. These may be indicators of depression. If you see signs of depression, contact professional psychological and psychiatric help immediately. Do not put this off! Get help at once. If anti-depressants are prescribed, don't be surprised. They can be beneficial. The survivor's life, dreams, hopes, ambitions and abilities have been devastated and they've lost more than you will ever understand. I wasn't depressed when I came home, but neither was I motivated to pick up projects that had been dormant since before my stroke. My lack of motivation was very unlike my pre-stroke behavior, but I couldn't get revved up chasing an old goal. My values and priorities have changed.

There are so many variables for stroke survivors that it's impossible for me to provide hard and fast guidelines to help you decide when help is needed. Stroke causes such a wide array of impairments that every survivor is unique physically and psychologically. Does the survivor function at a high level mentally and physically? Is the survivor physically impaired from the stroke? Is the survivor cognizant of what happened to them? Are they fully aware? All of these things and many more can have a bearing on the psychological health of the survivor. It seems particularly tragic to me that a person can survive stroke and brain damage and return home to commit suicide. The stroke experience is terrifying. Talk with the survivor about their experience. Invite them to talk about it. What have they learned? The more you learn, the better. When working with a survivor, do not treat them like a child, or use "special voices". This pandering is so demeaning, and inconsiderate, it makes my blood boil.

Today I still feel blessed for my stroke experience, as though I'm living in a state of grace and in perfect alignment with the universe. It's like I'm taking a test and God is whispering the answers in my ear. I believe Zen Buddhists call what I'm experiencing Satori. Satori is individual enlightenment that happens in a flash of sudden awareness and intuitive experience, traditionally gained through personal experience. My enlightenment began when I was spontaneously healed while leaving the history museum in Minneapolis. I felt the hand of God that day and I still feel giddy from the experience. It's like being in love. If I let go, I feel I might float into the sky. This psychological lightness is joyful and exhilarating. I'm filled with a love for every living thing. Because God made everything perfect and I love God, I love everything. I won't break out into song and dance, but it may end tomorrow. I hope this delicious feeling never ends, because it's wonderful. Answers to questions that have troubled me for years just pop into my head, and suddenly I know the unknowable. This first happened when I wanted to find Miss-Right after leaving the hospital. I had every intention of keeping my promise to God as an act of contrition if nothing else. Humility is good for the soul. Suddenly, I knew where to find her, and with dead certainty I knew exactly what I had to do. Every day is a precious miracle. I feel energy flowing through me like electricity and when I do, it never fails to trigger a laugh, because the feeling is so joyous and wonderful. This is how I felt as a kid, happy to be alive and right with the world. The idea that God made everything perfect came to me in a flash of enlightenment. I'd been wondering for weeks if animals make mistakes, so I studied Kato to see if she made any. She does, rarely. Unlike people, animals don't have myriad options and aren't motivated by jealousy, envy, greed, lust, or avarice, reasons many people get into trouble. Animals are limited to their normal, natural behavior and seldom surprise. Their every action must be what God intended. If this is true, every animal is a perfect manifestation of God, no matter its genus and phylum. Even the vampire bats, jungle snakes, leeches, scorpions, and fire ants I encountered in the tropics were perfect. My reasoning may lack Socratic precision, but I'm dead certain I'm right. I'm just not bright enough to construct the perfectly reasoned argument.

I live off a military pension and live modestly in my own apartment, cooking all my meals, doing laundry, doing the dishes, making up my bed, paying bills and doing everything independent life requires. I don't live in total penury but each month is a photo finish to see if food or money lasts longer. Don't think I'm complaining. I dug myself out of a pretty deep hole, and I've come further than I thought possible. Today, I'm happy to report there is life after stroke. Better still, the tweety birds have stopped flying around my head. Each survivor should allow ample time to realize what the lasting effects of their injury will be.

We can never know why bad things happen to us. Bad things happen to everyone. The Greeks created mythologies to explain the vagaries and seeming unfairness of life. One legend I've always enjoyed is that of Sisyphus. He was condemned by his Gods to a life of endless toil and useless struggle because he scorned them. It was Sisyphus's punishment to push a boulder up a mountain until he reached the top, where the boulder would roll down the other side. Then Sisyphus had to go to the bottom and push the bolder back up again, where the boulder always rolled down still again. This up down cycle was repeated endlessly. Some people have found inspiration, nobility and dignity in the travails of Sisyphus. "The struggle itself toward the heights is enough to fill a man's heart. One must imagine Sisyphus happy."[17] I've seen a metal representation of Sisyphus as a stick figure pushing a huge outsized metal boulder sitting on people's desks that I like. Some days I feel like Sisyphus because stroke rehabilitation is so challenging and difficult. There is a magnificence in Sisyphus' doggedness and refusal to give up that I feel is an important lesson for us all.

Another Greek legend I enjoy is that of the Moirai or Fates, three goddesses who were credited with controlling the birth, destiny and death of each person. Klotho spins the thread of each life. Lachesis allocates good and bad to each life, often with an undertone of sadistic cruelty. Atropos cuts the thread of life and we die. The Greeks felt the deck of life was stacked against us by the capricious and arbitrary acts of the fates. To battle against such unseen forces makes our infrequent victories that much more brilliant and meaningful. I was never a fan of mythology in school, but I've reached a point in my life where I understand the wisdom of myth. It is the challenges and trials in life that build our character and define our quality as people. If there were no difficulties to be overcome then where would we find the joy of achievement? It matters not at all that others cannot see what I've done, cannot know the distance I've come or understand the obstacles I've had to surmount. I know, and that is enough. I did not do these things for others, I did them for me alone, and I found great pride and satisfaction in the process. So will you. Do not despair. To struggle and win is priceless.

When I meet other survivors I often congratulate them on their recovery and their hard work without knowing exactly how they were effected by their stroke. I do this because all survivors had to be brave, all faced challenges that seemed impossible, and all survivors have worked very hard to get where they are. There is nobility in each struggle and each survivor deserves to be congratulated for their valiant achievement. No one can ever know what the survivor went through or the depths of their hell. It is enough just knowing they survived and prospered.

We all get frustrated when things don't break our way. A sign of my recovery is my ability to get angry. It's more than a year since my stroke and I'm just now able to get angry at the trivial irritants that plague everyone. This is a good sign, because it means my ego, my sense of self, is rebuilding. I like it. I don't like getting frustrated or upset, but I think this is a healthy sign after a year long hiatus. The love in my heart and my ability to finally get angry may seem to be at odds, but I seem to be able to be angry and feel love simultaneously. This is a new dimension for me, something I've never done before. When this happens, all I can do is laugh.

I suspect stroke survivors often suffer from post traumatic stress disorder. Studying PTSD should prove helpful. If there was one area where my stroke rehabilitation fell short, it was survivor psychology. Certainly I had psychologists and psychiatrists to talk with, and I did, but not in a focused, organized way. I think most survivors go through predictable stages of recovery. Without someone to lead the survivor through them, they are left to stumble and stagger through the recovery process on their own. This is stressful, and important stages of the recovery may be neglected. Dr. Kubler-Ross did a terrific job identifying specific and necessary stages of grieving. Why can't something similar be done for stroke recovery? Stroke can be a very traumatic experience. My stroke experience was reminiscent of my two years combat experience. I had undiagnosed PTSD when I came home from the war. More is known about PTSD today. We should use all our knowledge.

CHAPTER 15

POSSIBLE IMPAIRMENTS FROM STROKE

I originally planned to separate impairments by hemisphere of injury. Injury to the right hemisphere of the brain can cause certain impairments different from stroke injury to the left hemisphere of the brain. Specific impairments are determined by the exact location and severity of the injury. The more specific I tried to get, the more confusing it became. What follows are possible impairments that may occur as a result of stroke. The American Stroke Association and the American Heart Association occasionally separate impairments by hemisphere. If that would be helpful, give them a call using their free help line phone number found in the Resources for Families and Caregivers chapter and ask them to send the information you want.

My attempts to separate impairments by hemisphere were frustrating, confusing, and a perfect demonstration of brain damage at work. I had a heck of a time. Janine Reder, my wonderful speech language pathologist tried mightily to straighten me out, but I'm brain damaged. Here then are possible impairments as a result of stroke.

FIELD CUT Stroke often effects the vision center in the brain. Field cuts are fairly common. I have a left field cut and can see forward just fine but not to my left. My field cut prevents me from driving. Additional scanning is the only compensation. Field cuts rarely heal or disappear entirely but therapies are becoming available that hold a hint of promise. This is the most limiting impairment from my stroke. I cannot drive safely and must scan constantly to prevent collisions with furniture, solid objects, my cat, and other people. Things seem to pop up suddenly and surprise me when I bump into them or people suddenly appear as if they rose up out of the floor. This was pretty creepy for me at first.

POOR SHORT-TERM MEMORY I often write things down to compensate for this problem. This takes discipline but works well. I surprise myself constantly when I discover I've already done something I'm doing again. I forget things constantly. I forget conversations a lot, making those I communicate with very frustrated. If I put something down someplace, I forget where, so I misplace things often. This is one of my most irritating impairments. I forget I'm cooking, doing laundry, or set the phone aside while speaking with someone and then forget I was in the middle of a conversation. This gives people fits. Another problem associated with my memory is I can't remember if I've taken my meds for the day. This could have serious consequences so I've established a routine I follow closely to prevent an accidental re-dosing. When I arise every day, I lay out my meds for the day. Later, if I see them sitting there, I know I haven't taken them yet. This seems too simple but it works well because otherwise I can't remember if I've already taken my meds or not. Two weeks ago I bought a coconut cream pie and forgot it. By the time I found it, the pie had turned into that rare fourth state of matter. It wasn't a solid, it wasn't a liquid and it wasn't a gas, but it smelled like a petroleum refinery.

POOR ATTENTION SPAN This, coupled with my poor memory, is very troubling. Complex instructions, films and books are difficult for me to follow, so I lose interest quickly. I've read several books since my stroke, but each was a trial by fire. Information seems to register on my brain one drop at a time. There is no connectedness from one scene to another in films or from one sentence to another in books. Without any flow, things are disjointed, as if I'm snatching random information out of the air. Films are often just a random series of images that don't mean a thing. This steals the joy from films and books.

ERRATIC CONVERSATION I used to drive my friends and family nuts. In conversation I'd jump from one subject to another like a flea on a hot skillet. I thought I was doing fine, but later people told me I was jumping around and difficult to follow, so if this happens to your survivor, be patient. Chances are good this will disappear in time.

PARALYZED OR WEAK SIDE OF THE BODY Physical therapy may be necessary to regain full functionality. Determination and grit help.

DISORIENTATION, SPATIAL, AND PERCEPTUAL PROBLEMS make it easy for us to lose our way, fail to recognize landmarks, and get disoriented in simple situations. If you show a survivor the way to the store or someplace visited frequently, take your time and move slowly to make certain the survivor has the landmarks locked in their brain. Walking the back trail is also a helpful. The last thing anyone wants is for the survivor to get lost and become disoriented. Having done it many times, I know being lost is a terrifying experience. I always feel foolish and stupid when it happens to me. When possible, I take familiar routes to and from my destination. Now that I know the landmarks, there's nothing to it, unless I space out and forget to pay attention. When I suddenly wake up, I don't recognize a thing and I'm lost again. I did it again just yesterday on a route I've taken many times. When I walk the ground ripples, so I must move more slowly even though I know the ground is solid.

No Sense of Time Flow or Continuity Day to Day For me, the days don't feel connected for some reason. The normal flow of time, one day to the next, is gone. When I awaken, I seldom know if it is seven o'clock in the morning or evening. This is very confusing. Time can seem to drag slowly for us too. A **Digital watch with day/date functions** is very helpful when dealing with time issues. I never know the day or date, so a watch with these features makes life much easier.

Dysphagia (dis-FA-ge-ah) The inability to swallow food or drink. Sixty-five percent of stroke survivors have problems with this.[18] A speech therapist can teach the survivor to swallow properly so they can maintain good nutrition. Proper diet is a significant problem for survivors with dysphagia. Professional therapy is often required. See Speech Therapy on p. 107.

Organizational Problems, Sequencing or Multi-tasking Too many things to do at once gets me flustered and I can't think straight. Trying to do too much at once leaves me scatterbrained. Yesterday I forgot to put on a belt when I dressed for the day. I thought about it, but I got distracted and forgot all about putting on my belt.

I walked to town, about 2 miles away and then back home, after I ran some errands. I had to hold my pants up with one hand the whole way. Aside from feeling like a complete dope, it was a nuisance and robbed much of the joy from my otherwise pleasant walk.

COGNITIVE PROBLEMS I have great deal of difficulty understanding and following complex instructions. The instructions for a camera, a clock radio, programming a new telephone or instructions for any new equipment leave me angry and terribly frustrated. I don't have the patience or brain power to be successful. I try, but must wait for someone's help.

DIFFICULTY DRESSING PROPERLY This sounds silly but I have a heck of a time figuring out clothes. I know how they should be, but I have a tough time getting them on right. I've worn my clothes inside out or backwards many times and had to be told. I can feel something is wrong, but I'm lost figuring out what it is. They feel wrong, but look alright. A shirt or jacket not on a hangar looks like a wad of fabric, nothing more. I can't tell where to grab it to find the top or bottom. It should be embarrassing walking around looking like I dressed with my eyes closed, but I accept it because I'm doing the best I can. This happens more often than I'd like to admit.

I'M SOMETIMES ILLOGICAL This can be frustrating for people who argue with me. They must feel like they're arguing with Satan. When I think I'm right, I stick by my guns. Arguing with us to prove you're right or trying to always have the last word is childish. You won't like it. I don't always get my way, so why should you?

QUICK IMPULSIVE BEHAVIOR STYLE I don't have the patience I wish I did sometimes. Since I've always been impulsive, I seem to be normal in this regard.

STRUGGLE WITH NUMBERS Simple math, telling time and making correct change throw me. Numbers don't make sense to me. I know what numbers represent, but they make my skin crawl. Coming from a design and engineering background, this is the complete opposite of my former self. Numbers used to be my friends, and I was comfortable with them, so I can't fathom this cruel joke. With time this has abated slightly.

EMOTIONAL LABILITY Also called reflex crying, this is a tearful over-reaction. Crying comes on suddenly at inopportune times, often unheralded. This is most evident when I think of something personally sad. It's embarrassing, but what can I do? Guys aren't known for their crying jags, particularly out here in cow country. My horse used to go walleyed when it happened. I was trained from birth to never cry. Since I no longer wear triangular pants, and my lability has passed, I'm sorta regular now. Lability is a very common effect of stroke and may last for years.

Poor Decision Making Ability I've got to admit I've made some bone-headed decisions that I wish I hadn't. I've made decisions that impacted my life in a negative way. Sometimes I simply can't make a decision and kinda vapor lock and do nothing.

Difficulty Understanding Visual Cues This plays havoc with me when I'm getting dressed, putting clean sheets on my bed, or folding laundry.

LOSS OF MUSICAL ABILITY I used to enjoy playing the guitar. Though I wasn't what you'd call a prodigy before my stroke, I haven't attempted to play since and I have to trust the experts. Dexterity may be a problem and whistling is still a problem because my lips can't pucker properly for a decent whistle. With a broken pucker, brass and woodwind instruments could be problematic. Keeping the correct meter may also effected

DIFFICULTY FOLLOWING FAST-PACED ACTION ON SCREEN is a problem. I'm slow and my brain simply can't keep up, no matter how hard I try. I hate it, but there it is. I seldom go to films for this reason. I miss so much of a film, there's no point.

LOSS OF INHIBITIONS Experts say this happens in social situations where a survivor may blurt out something embarrassing or inappropriate.

FATIGUE is a problem for many survivors Stroke really takes a lot out of a person. Often we just don't have the energy or the reserves we once did. Consequently, we tire more easily and sleep more. Many survivors like myself nap during the day. Some days a cat-nap is all I need. Other days I'll sleep for three, four, or five hours.

ATTENTION TO DETAIL I went to the grocery store recently and bought a whole chicken to make chicken soup. Unfortunately, I neglected to check the "Sell by" date. I put him in the refrigerator when I got home and forgot it. A week later, when I pulled him out to make soup, he made my eyes water. He was a bit sour. That was the strongest chicken I've ever seen. He could've pulled a six- bottom plow down Main Street. My background is design engineering and details used to be my life, so I'm retraining myself to pay attention to details. I make mistakes, but mistakes are the price of learning.

I was watching a psychologist on TV today. He was talking about language skills developing on the left side of the human brain. As he spoke about the left side of the brain, he kept poking the right side of his head. I didn't know what to think. *Is he trying to trick me?* The disconnect between his words and his actions was troubling. Stuff like this happens all the time and drives me crazy. "The devil is in the details," to quote an architect whose name I've forgotten. He was dead right.

SPEECH AND LANGUAGE PROBLEMS See speech therapy p. 107.

PARALYSIS OR WEAKNESS This may disappear with physical therapy. New promising therapies are being developed, but rehabilitation can be a long and difficult journey.

Chapter 16

Resources for Families and Caregivers

If you are a new caregiver for a stroke survivor, you'll need all the courage, patience, understanding, and tolerance you can muster for the task ahead. Taking charge of someone else's life isn't easy. You have your own concerns, and now the patient's as well. Dividing your efforts can be physically and psychologically exhausting. When you have problems, and you will, contact the resources listed here and use their broad range of experience and expertise. They can help. Despite your best efforts, you may still have some guilt and stress because you can't possibly do everything that needs doing. The patient will lose some life satisfaction when they lose control of their life. Knowing they are no longer in control of their life is terribly demoralizing for the patient. The burden of stroke is difficult for everyone in the family; husbands, wives, children, siblings, and parents included. No one will have an easy ride, and each person must make adjustments for the new burden. Ultimately, some of your sacrifices will go unnoticed and unacknowledged. Be certain you take care of yourself, your family and your marriage. No matter how able, caring, giving, loving, and selfless you are, you aren't a super-hero with superpowers. You're flesh and blood, and extraordinary. Don't beat yourself up for things you can't help. Don't listen to neighbors, relatives, or anyone else concerning "what you should do." Listen to your heart and let it be your guide.

Krames Communications for speech difficulties
    Call free 1-800-333-3032

American Stroke Association for stroke problems
    Call free 1-888-478-7653

Stroke Family Warmline For Life After Stroke
    Call free 1-800-553-6321

BRAIN These people are involved in research
    Call free 1-800-352-9424

American Speech-Language-Hearing Association
    Call free 1-800-638-8255

National Rehabilitation Information Center
    Call free 1-800-346-2742

COURAGE STROKE Network for stroke problems
   Call free 1-800-553-6321

National Stroke Association for stroke problems
   Call free 1-800-787-6537

The Brain Injury Association for family help
   Call free 1-800-444-6443

American Heart Association for behavioral
   changes Call free 1-800-242-8721

National Institutes of Health Neurological Institute

   Call free 1-800-352-9424

Chapter 17

Wishful Thinking

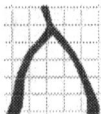

Ask, and it shall be given;
Seek, and ye shall find;
Knock, and it shall be opened.
Everyone that asketh, recieveth;
he that seeketh, recieveth;
To him that knocketh it shall be opened.
Matthew 7:7,8

Wishful thinking is a way to use your mind to get just about anything you want. Want better health? Want a better marriage? Want to earn more money? Want to be more happy? Want your dog to stop crapping on the floor? Want the best looking garden on your block? Want to save thousands of dollars and fix your own teeth free? Everyone wishes for something. I've no idea what your wishes may be, but if you do what I'm about to tell you, you can make most of your wishes come true with very little effort. Ah, there's the rub. To make your wishes come true, some effort is required, so this isn't exactly a free ride.

Every animal, fish, or fowl, conserves energy whenever possible. No living thing expends energy unnecessarily. When people conserve energy instead of doing what they should, they're lazy or lack motivation. Some people are afraid they might work too hard. What tragedy. Some spend more energy avoiding work than if they actually worked. Others try to fool the boss, and work hard at looking like they're working. The chronically lazy can die of thirst while sitting on a pile of shovels, because they're too lazy to dig for water. If you're super lazy, just ignore what I'm about to suggest, because it will require one or two minutes of effort each day to make your wishes come true. Because wishful thinking saved my life, I'll take a chance and spill some ink on it here. You'll probably think I'm mental when you read about it, but in the past year I've used wishful thinking to clarify my stroke fogged brain, cured prostate cancer, cured congestive heart disease, and fixed my own teeth. If wishful thinking hadn't done all this, I'd be skeptical too. Now that I've seen the power of the mind, and wishful thinking, I know it works. I don't know how it works, but it does. I don't know how my television works either. I couldn't build one to save my life. When I want to watch something, I just turn it on and watch. It's that simple. I won't try to convince you that wishful thinking works. This isn't a pitch. Because I used it successfully to clarify my mind and regain lost abilities, I'm going to tell you about it. Some people spend big bucks to learn this stuff. Wishful thinking worked for many of the things I've tried it on, but not all. Even though I'm not religious, I usually say a short prayer at the beginning and end of each "session." It can't hurt and I believe it helps. Here is how I cured myself of dis-ease. Each morning when I awaken, I perform my morning ablutions and sit in a comfortable chair, relax and cross my ankles in front of me. Next, I cross my wrists in front of me and twist my arms so my palms are facing one another. In this position interlace the fingers of both hands. Got it? This "knot" position is a fast and easy shortcut to your subconscious. If you cannot get into this position, you can use self-hypnosis, meditation or contemplation instead. The "knot" posture is much faster and easier than the relaxation process necessary for self-hypnosis, meditation or contemplation, so I use it exclusively. Once you've tied yourself in a knot, recite your wish or wishes aloud or mentally. I made a list of thirty or forty wishes, so I recite each wish the same way every morning and every evening. If a wish doesn't seem to be getting results, I change the wording of my wish slightly. Sometimes a wish doesn't "feel" right, so I'll change the wording slightly. A wish must be accepted by your subconscious in order to work. I begin each session with this prayer; "Oh God, hear my prayers and manifest my wishes." I close each session with this prayer; "I Thank You God for the blessings You have given me."

I've read and heard many theories on why wishful thinking works, but none of them agree, so I don't think anyone knows, including me. Here is my current theory. Each person's subconscious is programmed by the world around us. For example, when I was about four years old, Mrs. Bera, a neighbor lady, came over to see my mom. While they were talking, Mrs. Bera complained about not being able to sleep on her new hair do. When my mom suggested she sleep on her back, Mrs. Bera said, "Oh, I can't do that. I always have nightmares when I sleep on my back." Those words have stuck in my head and for the past fifty five years and I've never been able to sleep on my back. I don't worry about nightmares. I can't sleep on my back because I feel uneasy. The women didn't know I was eavesdropping and wouldn't have cared if they had, but when Mrs. Bera came out with that nightmare business she accidentally programmed my subconscious. This is an example of how easily everyone can be programmed unintentionally. Once our subconscious hears something, it may or may not believe it. The problem is we don't know what our subconscious may have picked up over the years. I sometimes do things for reasons I can't explain. Some of the things I do are not in my best interest, so I actually seem to be working against myself sometimes. Wishful thinking is a tool you can use to program your subconscious on purpose, so it's working for you, and not against you. The subconscious seems to have a hotline to God, so our prayers and wishes are answered pronto if we use a wish statement our subconscious will accept.

Doctors and medical science have known about the power of the mind for centuries because they've had plenty of evidence that the mind is a powerful ally in the treatment process. Mesmer is the earliest doctor I'm aware of who used the patient's mind as an ally through hypnosis in the seventeen hundreds in France to heal the patient.

Consider the lowly placebo. A placebo is a harmless sugar pill that is given to patients instead of real medicine. The patient is told what the medicine will do for them, and sometimes the patient is told what side-effects the medicine causes. In most studies, the placebo is as effective as actual medicine. What's more, the patient taking the placebo often has the same side-effects as a patient taking the real drug. This has been observed for centuries in countless medical trials, and it's generally known collectively as "the placebo effect." It clearly demonstrates the power of the mind to manifest symptoms it could not possibly have and the power of the mind to heal the body with nothing more than the lowly sugar pill. The key ingredient in many cures is the human mind. Unfortunately, most doctors know very little about enlisting the help of the patient's mind as an active ally. Wishful thinking enlists the mind as a willing accomplice in gaining what the practitioner desires.

The first step in wishful thinking is developing good wish statements.

How to make a good wish statement:

1) Make your wish present tense, not future tense.

2) Make your wish in first person.

3) Make your wish positive and free of negatives.

Follow these simple rules to make your wishes work. As I said, I made lists of wishes that fall into these categories:

1) I have one list of Health wishes.

2) I have another list of Wealth wishes.

3) I have a list of Well Being wishes.

4) I have a Bootstrap list that increases wish power and efficiency.

Make new categories if it's helpful to organize your wishes. I have perhaps ten or fifteen wishes of each type, so I have one sheet of Health wishes, one sheet of Wealth wishes, one sheet of Well Being wishes, and a final sheet of Bootstrap wishes. Your wishes must be specific. It helps if you can visualize the cause of a problem and visualize what needs to happen for your wish to come true. For instance, after my stroke, my brain was scrambled and my thinking was confused, so the first wish I made was "I make new neural pathways to clarify my thinking and improve my mental focus." While reciting this wish I visualized an old-fashioned telephone switchboard with all the wires being plugged in and properly connected. I had difficulty repairing my left field cut because I didn't know how my brain processed visual information or how it was disrupted by my stroke so I didn't know what to visualize to fix it. A general wish "My vision is healed, and I see perfectly well." isn't specific enough to get a cure. Visualization and specificity help tremendously.

Books are available with various wish statements you may want to help you make your wishes. A lady named Louise L. Hay has written a wonderful small, inexpensive handbook titled "Heal Your Body." This little booklet is full of wish statements that can be used as is, or modified for all sorts of specific health problems. You can get a copy from her website: **www.hayhouse.com** I've found wishful thinking works well for me on personal health issues, so Louise's book may be just what you need to improve your own health.

HERE ARE SOME SAMPLE WISHES FOR HEALTH ISSUES. MODIFY THEM TO SUIT YOUR NEEDS:

My prostate is healthy, well, and shrinking every day.

My veins and arteries are clean, clear, and have no blockage.

I am at the peak of health and vitality.

My heart is strong and in perfect health.

My cavities repair themselves with healthy new growth.

I make new neural pathways and regain control of my left hand.

My pulse is slow and my blood pressure is low.

I always awaken refreshed and rested.

All these and better things now manifest in my life.

I am a perfect channel for God's love and grace.

HERE ARE SOME SAMPLE WISHES FOR WELL BEING. MODIFY THEM AS NEEDED:

I am charged with positive energy and vitality.

I am tranquil and serene every moment of every day.

I look for the good in everyone and everything.

I am luminous like a radiant pearl and reflect people's thoughts back at them.

I am happy and content with my life.

I am in tune with the world around me and living God's plan.

The world is filled with positive energy and happiness.

I replace my failure programming with success programming.

HERE ARE SOME SAMPLE WISHES FOR WEALTH. MODIFY THEM TO SUIT YOUR NEEDS:

It is right for me to have more money than I need.

Money is attracted to me and I accumulate wealth easily.

I am paid what I am worth.

I am a child of the universe and the universe will not let me want.

Money is my friend and flows to me in great abundance.

I am free of money problems and live a life of plenty.

Here are some sample BOOTSTRAP wishes to increase your power and efficiency:

My subconscious quickly and easily accepts my wishes.

My wishes are powerful and are quickly manifest for me.

Each day my wishes improve and grow more powerful.

My thinking mind and my subconscious mind communicate openly and often.

Don't waste your time using wishful thinking to change the behavior of other people. Because people have free will, efforts in this direction are often useless, so don't try to put the "whammy" on someone. We are all subject to the laws of karma, so be careful what you wish for. Remember, thought is action.

Animals are easily manipulated, as I discovered this when I changed Kato's behavior within minutes. She was surprised at herself and didn't understand why she was behaving differently. Her reaction to her new behavior was funny. Now she thinks her new behavior is normal.

I've been considering forming a group of wishful thinkers who meet once a week and wish for common goals. I think a group of people making the same wish is much more powerful than an individual making a wish. If your town gets hit with bad weather frequently, everyone might agree to use a wish like this: "My town is protected by an energy bubble that storms slide around and cannot enter." I've been told weather can be controlled, but I've not tried it. Who knows?

I read somewhere in my research that our senses of sight, hearing, and taste are the senses of the conscious mind. Our subconscious mind's sense organ is our skin. If this is so, we can communicate directly with our subconscious through our skin. If this is true, snuggling makes a lot of sense. It might mean each snuggler's subconscious is communicating with the other. Children like to snuggle. Lovers like to snuggle. Many people like to snuggle at times, because it's often comforting and somehow reassuring. People seem to need human touch to keep themselves on an even keel. Given all this, maybe my theory about subconscious communication through touch has some validity. It's just an idea I had, so give it some thought.

The human mind is such a wondrous thing, and there is much we don't know about it. Trying to figure out how and why it works is like trying to guess the identity of an unknown creature on the opposite side of a thick curtain from you by the bulge it makes as it leans against the curtain. If it were an elephant, you could probably tell the animal was big, but it could be a giraffe, a man on a ladder, an elephant, or any number of things. Simply based on limited evidence, it would be impossible to figure out what was causing the bulges you saw in the curtain. Wishful thinking is sorta like that. I know if we do certain things, we often get our wishes fulfilled, but I don't know why it works sometimes and not at others. No one does as far as I can tell. I'd been hearing about it for almost a year and always blew it off because I thought it couldn't possibly work. Then, when I was diagnosed with prostate cancer based on a series of biopsies, I was desperate and scared, so I finally tried it. Months later, I had a second series of biopsies. After they were analyzed, my doctor told me my cancer had disappeared. Yip, Yip, Yippie! Six months later I underwent a series of tests on my heart and my doctor told me I had congestive heart disease. I cranked up wishful thinking pronto and within a month I was told my heart condition had disappeared and my heart was working just fine with no trace of disease. These two instances are why I'm big on wishful thinking. I've cured bunches of lesser medical problems with it. One that I battled for almost forty years I healed in less than twenty four hours with wishful thinking, but these smaller issues were tiny nuisances compared to cancer and heart disease, so I don't mention them often. I'm relieved I was able to fix things that medical science hadn't been able to, but these smaller problems are less dramatic.

I know wishful thinking sounds screwy and like a bunch of crap. I felt exactly the same way until I used it with amazing results. If you're as skeptical as I was, and I imagine you are, I don't blame you. My problem is I know it works and I want to help people, but when I talk about it, people shake their head and start walking away mumbling to themselves. Wishful Thinking sounds impossible, but it works.

Suggested reading for Wishful Thinking concepts:

Better Health with Self-Hypnosis by Frank S. Caprio, M.D.

Creative Visualization by Shakti Gawain

Quantum Healing by Deepak Chopra, M.D.

AFTER WORD

A MIGHTY BIG RABBIT

In nineteen fifty one, when I was almost five years old, I was living with my family on the Washington Bar Ranch, a mixed horse, cattle, and sheep outfit in the Madison Valley, north of Yellowstone National Park in the Montana Rockies. I had an experience I've never discussed with anyone outside my family. While playing outside one day I saw a giant rabbit standing upright like a man less than twenty feet from me. He was as tall as my father, if you don't include the rabbit's ears, which altogether made him taller than anyone I'd ever seen. In aspect, he looked like the average rabbit but for his size and stance. I got excited and ran to him, but when he saw me coming, he fled and jumped over a pile of tailings I would guess was ten feet tall. He was incredibly fast and moved with such speed that I had no chance whatever of catching him. Tailings are mounds of rock and gravel mining spoil. There was an abandoned gold dredge on the ranch that made countless piles of tailings as it worked its way up North Meadow Creek searching for placer gold years earlier. I scrambled up the tailings as fast as I could go, and down the other side so I might at least see where he went. There, I found a large hole leading horizontally into a nearby drift of tailings. The hole was large enough for me to stand erect at the entrance. I was thrilled, and felt it must surely be the rabbit's home, so I walked inside to find him. Ten or fifteen feet into the tunnel, it petered out at a rock wall. I was stumped and couldn't understand how the rabbit had given me the slip. I was certain I had him trapped. Later, when I went home and reported the big rabbit to my folks, they burst out laughing. I knew rabbits weren't supposed to grow six feet tall, but I reported what I'd seen, none the less. I accepted the big rabbit with equanimity, as a matter of course. In a world filled with magic, a giant big rabbit fit right in. I don't know what I saw that day, but I've told you what happened as well as I'm able.

The rabbit on the cover was drawn by James Stewart, the actor, after the wonderful film "Harvey", in which he starred, was released. The film is about a big rabbit named Harvey that only Stewart's character Elwood P. Dowd can see. Dowd says Harvey is a Pooka, and comes from a place "where space and time have no objections." A Pooka is a playful shape shifter from Irish and Celtic mythology. In the film, Dowd's family wants him committed to a sanitarium because he sees a giant rabbit where others see nothing. The film was released in nineteen fifty, one year before my rabbit adventure. I didn't see or know of the film until I reached adulthood many years later. I used Mr. Stewart's sketch of Harvey on the cover as a reminder of the magic and mystery of life. When I searched for a cover theme, Mr. Stewart's sketch seemed absolutely perfect.

PIANO LESSONS

In nineteen fifty nine, when I was in the eighth grade, my mother enrolled me in piano lessons. I had no interest in piano, but I suppose she felt my rural Montana background had left me with a few rough edges, so when the edict came down, I dutifully took lessons from a teacher in my neighborhood. I was careful not to tell anyone at school about it. I thought piano lessons were sissy stuff, so I didn't say a word about them. I practiced on an old upright in the living room. It was no big deal, though I'd rather been out playing ball with the other guys instead of practicing scales. One day, I asked my teacher to teach me Liszt's Second Hungarian Rhapsody so I might have a dramatic show piece, something to showcase my "talents." This might seem like an odd choice, but at the time, rock 'n roll was still in diapers. Elvis, The Everly Brothers, Rick Nelson, The Platters, Perry Como, The Coasters, Bobby Darin, and Chuck Berry loomed large on the popular music landscape. The British invasion was yet to come. America was pretty square, I suppose. So was I. My teacher was teaching me to read music, but her instructions were like drops of water on my granite brain, and didn't make much impression. She liked my Hungarian Rhapsody idea and soon I was able to play the complex piece "by ear" flawlessly. Monkey see, monkey do. At the time, I attended frequent parties given by kids in my class. At most of these, someone would start banging on the piano. Nothing serious, just "chopsticks" "Heart and Soul" or feeble "Boogie Woogie", junk like that. One afternoon Mr. Popular, the class hero, had a party at his home, and sure enough, before long the popular kids were fiddling around on the piano. After they'd exhausted the tired junk we heard at every party, I took a seat at the piano, and announced I'd like to "give it a try." After a few catcalls and protests from the peanut gallery, I jumped into my showcase with zeal and verve. I finished my amazing performance with a sparkling flourish. Brother, when I was done, everyone was hanging on the ropes, knocked out! My classmates were astounded. Their compliments gushed and flowed like wine at a bacchanalia. It was a moment I'd planned for more than a year, and I reveled in their praise and astonishment. "Who was that masked man?" Everyone should have one moment like this in their life.

MEET THE BEATLES

In the spring of nineteen sixty three I was finishing my sophomore year of High School. My mom worked as a waitress at a nearby restaurant. Mrs. Myers, one of her customers had a daughter named Sharon, who was a budding singer/songwriter. Sharon had performed on local radio often and began recording for various record labels under the names Sherry Lee, Jackie Dee, and Jackie Shannon. After changing labels again, Sharon began recording as Jackie DeShannon. Sharon had a couple songs on the radio and she was a big deal for a local Batavia girl. Well, Mrs. Meyers mentioned to my mom that Sharon was going into Chicago to meet the Beatles when they flew into town for the first time. My mom told Mrs. Myers I was crazy about the Beatles, and I was, too. Beatles music was so different from anything else. It was revolutionary, and I was drawn to it like a moth to a yard light. Kids generally fell into one of two camps; one camp liked Elvis and old fashioned junk like that, but the other camp, my camp, was absolutely mad about the Beatles. Beatles music was a clarion call to most kids. It would be easier to make water to run up hill than convince Beatles fans that they weren't the living end. At school that year, we had a "talent show." In the show, three classmates and I lip-synced "She Loves You" and "I Want To Hold Your Hand" while we jumped around on stage wearing bad "Beatles" wigs, as girls from our class screamed hysterically on cue. It was pretty corny, but the illusion was made more convincing by the din and the chaos. In the audience, most adults were clueless, and many thought we were the genuine article. Well, Jackie's mom said, "If your son would like, he can come with us into Chicago and spend the day with the Beatles." When my mom told me about it, I just about flipped! Holy cats! Two weeks later, on a Saturday, the Beatles flew into Chicago, but I had a scheduling conflict and was trapped at my first piano recital. My mom worked hard for her money, and wanted to see what her money had gotten her, so she insisted I perform a little keyboard magic at the stupid recital and forget about the Beatles. I was crushed! At the recital I played an mistake-free French composition my father said was "girlish". It was bright and carefree, but I didn't care one way or the other. *I could be spending the day with the Beatles, and you want manly music too?*

It's ironic that the source of my solitary fleeting musical triumph was the cause of my greatest disappointment. Jackie DeShannon went on to tour two dozen cities with the Beatles and became a highly successful and much sought after songwriter. She was the <u>genuine</u> article. Hundreds of her songs have been recorded and performed by a pantheon of world famous performers. Hooray for Jackie! I'm sorry I missed it, but I was otherwise engaged at my first and final piano recital. I never played piano again.

The Last Hobo

After my discharge from the Army, I worked as a highway construction inspector in Illinois. One nice summer day I was "walking the job." We'd just finished resurfacing fifteen miles of rural highway, and I was walking all of it to make certain all the station numbers were in place. Traffic was sparse and my mindless job was simple, so I had lots of time to look around and enjoy the day. Up ahead of me I saw a man walking toward me on the same side of the highway as me. As he approached me, I could see he carried some sort of sack on his back. I was curious if he would say anything or simply pass by without a word. Because we were miles from anywhere and were the only two people in sight, I felt it was natural that we speak, but many people won't talk unless provoked. I didn't know if he would be tongue-tied or how he would react to meeting someone out in the middle of nowhere.

As we drew closer, we both smiled and said hello. Then we stopped standing face to face and started to converse. As we talked, I became intrigued by the old man with the gunny sack on his back. He was interesting. Soon, he started to walk past me and continue on his way, so I turned around and walked along with him, going back where I'd just come from. We walked and talked in that fashion for a mile or two until I learned his life story.

He was a hobo. He didn't ride the rails like hobos of the depression, but walked where he wanted to go. In the summers, he walked up through Illinois and Iowa. By the time fall came along and it was turning cold, he'd be down in Georgia or Florida where he would spend the winter months. Next summer, he'd work his way up into Illinois and Iowa again and repeat his circular migration like this, year after year. "Why do you do this? Don't you have a home?" I asked him. "I used to. I once had a wife and a home like everyone else. I was a structural engineer, until the pressure got to be too much. One day something in me just snapped and I had a nervous breakdown. My hands shook so hard that I couldn't keep coffee in a cup. I was sent to a nervous hospital. After being locked up and drugged for a while, I decided I didn't want to spend the rest of my life like that, so I escaped and started walking. I don't have problems with my nerves now, so this life suits me," he said. "How do you live? How do you eat?" I asked. I had a million questions I wanted to ask. I'd never met a hobo, and I was anxious to know how he survived and prospered. Everyone I'd ever known had homes and families and cars and jobs and bills and problems, but this man had none of the things we consider necessary for happiness, yet he was the happiest person I'd ever met, and healthier while having nothing than he was when he had everything. We walked on for another hour, and in that time he taught me how to survive without money or the baggage of modern society. I was amazed by his knowledge and ingenious survival techniques. He was a true ascetic, but unlike Sidhartha, he wasn't looking for enlightenment. He only wanted to be left alone so that he might find peace. He loved the world and knew exactly how he fit in. His gunny sack was full of plastic milk jugs and empty plastic bleach bottles. These were the raw materials for the pinwheels, paddlewheels and whirligigs he made to give kids he met along the way.

Santa Claus

Years later, I was still living in Illinois when I played Santa at an annual employee Christmas party. My white hair, white beard, and roundish shape made me a natural for the part. Talk about type casting! When I walked into the party dressed in a shabby Santa suit, all the three, four, and five year olds were so excited, and most were overcome with excitement. Santa was a superhero to those kids. Many didn't want a toy, though I had many to hand out. Most just wanted a hug, and anxiously held out their arms to me. I spent a lot of time giving hugs to those children. To feel accepted and loved by Santa was too much, and some just couldn't hold their water when they sat on my lap. Some kids would tug on my beard suspecting a fake, but when they found my beard was genuine, they were stunned, and forced to reconsider their suspicions.

GOOD FRIDAY

My dad was a Navy man. When I was a kid, he talked glowingly about sailing and I never forgot it. Years later, when my design work took me to North Carolina, I met people who sailed and often took me along. My dad was right, sailing is great fun. I liked it so much I joined the U.S. Power Squadron and took courses in seamanship, weather, boat handling sailing, and navigation. During those first two years I sailed everything I could, including craft up to fifty feet in length on Pamlico Sound. Part of becoming a competent sailor is learning the lingo. Sailing and sailboat terminology is like a foreign language, so the learning curve for a land lubber like myself was steep. My ultimate ambition was to be a blue water sailor, so I applied myself and worked hard. Blue water sailing is ocean sailing, more dangerous and unpredictable than inland, lake, or costal brown water sailing because help is often further away or nonexistent. The following summer, I bought a cutter rigged Catalina twenty two named "Good Friday." It wasn't the forty foot blue water boat I dreamed of, but the trim little Catalina was a good learning tool. Over the following year, I spent weekends sailing Good Friday on Pamlico Sound, out of Washington, North Carolina, where I had it docked. These were the sailing grounds of the notorious pirate and scoundrel Blackbeard, a.k.a. Edward Teach. East of there at Bath, North Carolina, Blackbeard owned property and was married. East across the sound is Okracoke Island, where Blackbeard was caught in 1718 by troops from Virginia and fought a furious battle. During the fray, Blackbeard sustained twenty sword wounds and five gunshot wounds before expiring. In a final act of contempt, the troops beheaded Blackbeard and threw his remains overboard. His head was tied to the bow sprit (the pointy part in the front) of his boat and sailed away as an object lesson to those who would defy British law. Blackbeard's death marked the end of the age of piracy.

As my skills improved and my confidence grew, I finally felt ready for ocean sailing. I'd been reading about it for years, so I had a good understanding of the risks and how to handle them. I asked a friend, Rick, from Illinois to join me for my first ocean sailing adventure. He had no sailing experience, so my proposal sounded like big fun. Ignorance is bliss. After Rick arrived, we loaded the food, fuel, water and navigation charts we'd need for our weeklong adventure onboard Good Friday. Early the following morning, we cast off. Yo ho ho and a dead man's chest. I was apprehensive because I knew the risks and hoped my skills and little boat were up to the challenge. Scared though I was, I didn't consider canceling our trip. I was determined to live my dream. As we headed out, my thoughts we consumed with a thousand details. Had I overlooked something? Would my ancient little kicker motor last? Would the navigation lights work alright for night sailing? Would the weather hold? I imagined all sorts of ugly endings for our trip and my little boat. Twenty two feet is not much boat under you on the open ocean, and I felt every inadequate foot of it as we sailed down the Intercoastal Waterway. Three days later, we arrived at Beaufort, North Carolina. The next morning, we sailed out Beaufort Inlet, past Shackleford Banks and were at last in the Atlantic Ocean. I was so apprehensive I could barely whisper. When the swells picked up, I gripped the tiller so tightly my fingers were numb. A short time later, we came upon four men in a tiny john boat bottom fishing. They were riding out the large swells as if it were nothing. I was amazed to see their tiny craft had just two inches of freeboard. Freeboard is the distance from the water to the top of the boat's sides where it would take on water and flood. Seeing those intrepid fishermen and their pitiful craft, I realized Good Friday had four feet of freeboard, and I began to relax somewhat. If those jaybirds weren't worried with two inches, I certainly wasn't going to worry with four feet. When we were out of sight of land, I took another look at my charts and confirmed our heading for Cape Lookout, which was our scheduled anchorage for the night. Rick made all the sail changes as we went along while I sailed and kept an ear cocked for weather reports on the radio. As we approached the Cape, a school of porpoise swam along side us, and individual porpoise took turns frolicking and playing in our bow wave. Blue water sailing is wonderful and everything I imagined it to be. The postcard blue sea, and the way sunlight streams down through the depths, was almost hypnotic. At the Cape, we dropped the hook and enjoyed a good meal, Jimmy Buffet music and good fellowship. I'd installed a good CD player and used to play Wagner's majestic "Ride of the Valkyrie" whenever I got in a good blow on the Pamlico. It was thrilling when Good Friday was pounding heavily, the wind was up, and spray was in the air. Gosh, that was great fun.

Three days after leaving Cape Lookout we sailed the final leg of our journey back up Pamlico Sound with banners flying. After we arrived at my marina, I finished tying off the spring lines just as the sun was setting. It was a good trip. All my early fears had been for nothing. Rick performed fine and would have made a great powder monkey in another age. The weather held, and I didn't blunder and sink us, so my first ocean adventure was wonderful. Nothing is so life affirming as facing a difficult challenge successfully, just as no one understands the value of freedom better than those who fought for it. I'd much rather try and fail than always regret not having even tried. History proves no worthy goal is ever gained without risk. I've always been a risk taker. Sometimes I win and sometimes I lose. My regrets aren't about my many losses; they're about only what I didn't try. Certainly, my sailing adventure was no nautical epic like Richard Henry Dana's "Two Years Before the Mast", or Rafael Sabatini's "Captain Blood", but it taught me that if we let it, fear makes prisoners of us all. Damn the torpedoes, full speed ahead.

SANTA CLAUS REDUX

Later that summer my brother came to visit, so I suggested we go out to Okracoke Island and spend the week there. Okracoke Island is a popular barrier island vacation spot because the island is largely untouched by civilization and is one of the few stretches of Atlantic coast "the way it used to be." We drove down to Swan Quarter and got in line for the next ferry. North Carolina has a wonderful ferry network. We stood beside my car as we waited with other vacationers for the ferry to arrive. As I stood there, off in the distance I heard a kid shout, "Hey, there's Santa!" Instead of cutting my white hair and my full white beard, I usually ignored kid's shouts. Dressed in cutoffs, running shoes, and a luau shirt, I looked like just another vacationer. When the ferry arrived, I pulled my car aboard and walked up to the top deck smoking lounge. When the ferry pulled away, I lit up and watched the waters of Pamlico Sound slip silently beneath us. The sound is a large, irregularly shaped body of water extending from Manteo, North Carolina near its northern point to Morehead City, North Carolina ninety miles away to the south. The sound is relatively shallow and roughly twenty to forty miles wide east to west, separated from the Atlantic Ocean by a thin string of low barrier islands on the east. This is hurricane country. The power and destruction of a large hurricane is difficult to comprehend unless you've been through one or two.

I find watching water, be it rivers, oceans or something smaller, very relaxing. Then, I felt something, and I looked down to see a small boy, perhaps five or six years old, tugging on my shirt. When I looked at him, he whispered up to me. "Are you Santa Clause?" he asked, just loud enough for me to hear. "Yes," I replied instantly. "What are you doing here?" he asked me in a whisper. Looking around, I saw a woman sitting near us in the lounge watching us closely. I felt she must be the boy's mother. She waited breathlessly, to see how I'd respond. "Well," I said, "I had a busy Christmas this year. There's lots to do at the North Pole, so I'm taking a vacation, just like you and your family." That made sense to him, so he turned to leave, but before he had gone, I said, "don't tell anyone I'm here." Like a shot, he was gone. His mom was laughing, and said to me, "You're in trouble now! That boy can't keep his mouth shut to save his life!" I wondered if maybe I'd started something I'd regret, but quickly put the boy out of my mind. Five or ten minutes later, the boy returned to the lounge and walked up to me grinning broadly. His smile made me suspect he'd blabbed. "Did you tell anyone I was here?" I asked him, worried things might spin out of control. Instantly he shook his head. "Good, good for you. Just for keeping my secret, I'm going to give you the best Christmas ever this year," I said to him, much relieved. His eyes grew large with surprise and wonder at my promise. After thinking for just an instant, my little co-conspirator whispered up to me, "Don't give the other kids anything." I paused for just a breath and said, "Alright. You have a merry Christmas." Away he ran again, happy and confident next Christmas was wired. I was afraid his mom would be upset, but she seemed to enjoy our exchange, because she laughed warmly. The boy's unabashed self-interest and quick thinking tickled me. I suspected he was the youngest in his family and often felt shortchanged. Even though Santa was in his corner, the little guy wanted a bases loaded grand slam homer of a Christmas, something no one would ever forget.

THE BLUE FISH

Late last summer I took Luke, my nephew's four year old son, fishing. He brought his toy kiddy rod along so he could fish too. Tied to the end of his line was a blue plastic fish that came with his little rod. When we got to the fishing hole, I grabbed my gear and quickly began catching fish, leaving Luke to his own devices. Later, I walked over to him to see how he was doing. I found him sitting on the riverbank dangling his blue plastic fish in the water. Curious, I asked him how he expected to catch a fish with no hook on his line. Luke said other fish would make friends with his blue fish and want to come home with us. I've never heard a more sweet, innocent, or warm hearted thought in my life.

THE STRANGER

The man who almost died of brain hemorrhage more than eighteen months ago and the man I am today are different people. My recovery has been agonizingly slow, but I continue to work for full recovery. I chose my title immediately after I was discharged from the VA Medical Center. When other stroke survivors hear my title, they will often give me a nod and a smile of understanding. Brain damage makes everything seem strange. But, more than that, my experience forced a painful reappraisal of my life and direction. I didn't like everything I saw, so I changed what I felt needed changing. As a result, I'm more compassionate, more tolerant, more accepting, more open, and more understanding of others, than ever before. Longtime friends are shocked by the changes they see in me, and have told me so. Many of them have had to become reacquainted with me. It seems weird, but it's necessary.

LIFE

I am amazed by the tenacity of life. Everywhere I look life flourishes, and once it gains a foothold, it hangs on and refuses to give up no matter how harsh the conditions or difficult that life may be. Even on frigid, windblown mountain tops of Montana I found life, desperately hanging on, struggling to survive, and unwilling to give up, quit, or die. It's amazing. In my driveway, growing from thin cracks in the concrete, volunteers live and survive, clinging to life in the most inhospitable conditions imaginable. I find this incredible. I've faced death many times, but I still hang on and want to live. There have been times when I wanted to give up, but when given the choice between death or life, I always choose life. Life is an endless struggle, as Sisyphus showed. No one said it would be easy, and it's not. Every plant or animal on the planet would rather live than die. I know this because in every instance they (we) struggle to survive. Actions speak louder than words. Fight for life as though it were precious. Life is a gift from God. Don't waste it.

COURAGE

If you have a loved one recovering from stroke or other traumatic brain injury, get them involved in their recovery. Don't allow them to cede their capabilities to brain damage without a heck of a fight. They will have to dig deep to find the strength they'll need to rehabilitate themselves. When things look hopeless, and the survivor feels like giving up, they'll need to get mad, and then get mean. Don't let brain damage win. Refuse, absolutely refuse, to give up. Recovery can be difficult and exhausting psychologically. There will be days when it seems as though improvement isn't possible. This is a trap. Don't fall for it. You and the survivor will need iron resolve to reach the recovery they're capable of. I was fortunate because Dr. Johnson suggested this book. It became my passion, and forced me to come to terms with what happened to me. I still feel my stroke was the best thing that ever happened to me. I gained more than I lost and I'm very grateful for it. My impairments preclude a return to design work. Friends encourage me to try, but I've lost too much and simply don't have the mental horsepower. Maybe I'll run away with the circus and give pony rides. That's about my speed.

KATO

I go fishing most days and always sing to Kato when I return. She loves me whether I've caught fish or not. I missed her something awful while I was in hospital. When I returned home, she was all over me and slept with all of her feet in the small of my back the first night. It was reassuring for both of us. She's lying on my feet as I write this, and I can feel her purring. It's 3:30 AM. She helps with all my writing. She's an American bob tail I found on a tobacco farm in North Carolina. She loves it when I stick a big toe in her ear and massage her gently.

178

Some things never change. May the blessings be. Tonight she was watching me as I finished making a sandwich I was particularly proud of. When I felt a rush of love and optimism, I said to her, "I think we're going to make it." We will too. I'm certain.

AN IMPORTANT LESSON

Today I went fishing. Along the way I saw a Swainson's hawk close by sitting on a fence post staring back at me. A Swainson's is a beautiful bird with dark brown feathers across its back and wings, and a cream colored chest and underbelly with dark speckles. It has a dark mask around it's head and eyes like Zorro. Ten minutes later, I watched a great horned owl fly to a landing in a tall cottonwood tree. Half an hour later, I watched a mature Bald Eagle soar above me, fishing, as I fished in the Heart River below. He gave a "skree" that echoed off the surrounding hills. I've been watching him for four years, since he was just a chick, first fledging out. I feel like a treed bear when I can't get out in nature. Nature is healing, restoring, and my patient teacher. In surroundings like this, my problems seem absolutely trivial. Never forget the sun is shining somewhere, and while it shines, there is hope. Guard your health as though it were a treasure. Your body is your vessel. It is the captain's job to see the vessel makes the journey safely. If the vessel is lost, it's cold comfort to know the captain had the right of way. Pride cannot replace good judgment

MAGIC

When people saw Mary Martin fly as Peter Pan many years ago, some saw only the wires that supported her, and took devilish delight in pointing them out, as though they might get extra credit. They couldn't see with childlike wonder, and insisted on destroying the illusion for others, so the effect was wasted on them, which is a shame, because they missed the whole point.

Remember in the Wizard of Oz when Dorothy was warned not to look behind the curtain? There are things we shouldn't know for our own good. If we look behind the curtain, who gains? If we see only the wires and none of the wonder, what have we lost? Many young children believe Santa exists. The idea of flying reindeer and a kindly generous fat man squeezing down their chimney with a bag of gifts seems perfectly reasonable. I'll not be the one who points out the wires, because I remember vividly what it was to see as a child sees with a child's eyes. I remember the joy and wonder and rightness of the world. I refuse to see boogie men and hide under my bed at the mention of magic. Some people see dark sinister forces at work at the mention of the word. These mealy-mouthed sob-sisters make me tired. They've forgotten their innocence and what it was to see with innocent eyes. Help others and pray often. Don't look for evil. You'll find it. There will always be something to complain about if you must.

A JOURNEY NOT FOR NOTHING

Thankfully, my lability is now a thing of the past. I haven't had a good cry in over a year, but I gotta tell ya, when I watch an old movie, and the good guy gets the girl, or the underdog wins over impossible odds, or someone's family gets the help they need just in the nick of time, or a woman perseveres and finds success after great sacrifice, I get a little misty eyed. It's no accident that the universal theme of triumph over adversity has been cherished since the time of the Greeks because, if we're lucky, we see it in life around us. If I had my life to live over, I'd find the sweetest woman I've ever known and, if she'd have me, I'd never let her go. No amount of wishing can change the past, but my mistakes weren't for nothing. Through them, I learned a great deal. I learned a sweet disposition and a kind heart are qualities more valuable than beauty or wealth. Beauty fades, and money spends, but a sweet disposition and a kind heart are forever.

STORY TELLING

Because I'm half Scots-Irish and half Cherokee, story telling is in my blood. We preserve our history and teach important lessons with stories. Stories have been important to my ancestors since they were painting themselves blue. If you don't believe what I've told you about meeting God, wishful thinking or chasing a giant rabbit, I wouldn't be a bit surprised, because it's natural to doubt things strange and marvelous. When Lewis and Clark invited the chiefs of the plains tribes to Washington to meet President Jefferson and see the sights, those who went beheld wonders beyond their comprehension. When they returned to their tribes and told what they'd seen, they were doubted, vilified and considered mad. Chief Sheheke and other great chiefs simply couldn't make their stone-age cultures understand the wonders of an emerging industrial society. When Moses reported a burning bush that spoke to him, I suspect he had a few doubters in his audience too.

MY BLUE CAP

In the chapter titled "A Recognition Lesson" I explained my hard-headedness. This is a tale of the reverse. The year before my stroke, I was working for a company in Billings, Montana. One day, Dana, my manager made a big deal out of presenting me with a company ball cap at a department meeting as a "reward" for something or other. It was a good cap, but I didn't care for the dark green color. After the meeting broke up, I went to a different department and spoke with the manager there. When I asked if he had any company caps, he reached down and pulled a dark blue ball cap from his desk and without any ceremony, tossed it to me. Except for the color, it was identical to the green one. Both had our company logo in white across the front. The next morning, I carried both hats to work and put them in the large bottom drawer of my desk before anyone else arrived. At first, I wore the green cap around the office, thinking I might learn to like the color. Soon, Dana arrived, and we began opening the store for the day. Just as we started, Randy, a buddy in my department, arrived and gave us a hand. When we were done, I sat down at my desk and made a few phone calls. While I was fiddling around, I decided I really didn't like my green cap much, and I decided to change to the blue one. I leaned down behind my desk, and quickly swapped the green for the blue. I was done in a flash. When I sat back up, I noticed Randy, staring at me from across the office, but I didn't give it much thought. Ten or fifteen minutes later, for no particular reason, I changed hats again. When I sat back up, I saw Randy do a double take. I wondered about it, but that was all. I kept changing hats all morning, when the mood struck me. I don't know why, but I had no reason not to change caps. Just before lunch, Randy slipped over and stood in front of my desk. "I thought Dana gave you a green cap," he said, studying my blue cap like I had a Yeti sitting on my head. For some reason, he seemed suspicious of my cap. "He did," I replied casually, ignoring Randy's odd theatrics. When he leaned across my desk to within inches of me, I detected the sweet scent of opportunity. "Maybe it's the light in here," he said, "but I could swear your cap looks blue." "Blue?" I asked in shocked disbelief. "You're color blind!" I accused. "No, I don't think so," Randy replied, with a hint of concern in his voice. "Maybe you should have your eyes checked," I suggested paternally. It was tough keeping a straight face and reining in the laughter that threatened to explode from me, because Randy thought my blue cap was green but looked blue. "I hate this color, but Dana said green was all he had," I added, corroborating one lie with another. "I don't know what it is, but your cap looks blue," Randy said, pinching his face into a muscular squint like Popeye. "It may look blue, but it's still nasty green," I replied dismissively. I kept changing caps all day, at random intervals, and secretly watched Randy's reaction. Sometimes he'd shake his head, as if his wiring was bad and could be fixed with a good smack. At other times, he'd rub his eyes, like he was scrubbing dirty windows. My stifled laughter nearly escaped several times, but I always managed to keep a straight face and swallow it down. As the day wore on, Randy grew more drawn and haggard, and looked about ready to check himself into the nearest hospital. I didn't tell anyone about my prank. Who would believe it? It seemed impossible that someone would doubt their own eyes. At five o'clock, our quitting time, I was walking out to my truck, when Cindy, Randy's girlfriend, arrived to carry him home. Soon, Randy walked out to meet her. Maybe it was my imagination, but I thought his walk looked a little wobbly and unsteady. When Randy got into Cindy's car, I paused to watch from a distance while he explained his vision troubles to her. As I was getting into my truck, I saw Cindy staring at me or my blue cap. I waved a hello and quickly buckled up. If body language is any indicator, they were arguing when I drove away. Looking back on it, my prank worked because Randy never saw me make a swap, and he didn't know I had two caps. When my cap inexplicably changed color, he suspected something was wrong with his eyes. The more frequently it happened, the more confounded and adrift he became. The following day, I showed Randy both my caps. He was surprised and relieved, happy his eyes were healed. I knew he felt like a dope, and he knew I knew he felt like a dope, but I didn't rub it in. That would be cruel.

A PROMISE KEPT

I've told you about my need to find a former love and apologize for my shabby behavior. Three months after my discharge from hospital, my nephew carried me two thousand miles so I could. This is what happened. I went to the home where she lived when we were dating in nineteen sixty five, and nervously knocked on her door. I felt like I was going to the wood shed for a much belated whipping, but I forced myself to put one foot in front of the other and keep moving, despite my shame and guilt, and wouldn't allow myself to stop until I reached her door. I was determined to pay off on my promise to God. Wild horses couldn't have pulled me away. She wasn't home, but her sister was. It was a very emotional moment for me when I walked into her home after a forty year absence. I tried to explain myself, but my lability kicked in and I couldn't stop crying. Between my sobs, my tears, and my choked voice, I was just about incomprehensible.

In hindsight, it was a pretty funny scene. I didn't explain my lability or mention I was recovering from a stroke, because I was afraid I'd look like I was fishing for sympathy, when all I wanted was five or ten minutes to say my piece to someone who wasn't home. I fought to regain my composure and rein in my raging emotions, but I was such a mess it was impossible, so I decided to just shut up and not say anything more. It wasn't a wasted trip though, because her sister told me my former love had two daughters and was happy. Just the rumor of her happiness made my trip worth it. Her sister asked for my phone number so she could call, if she wanted, but she never did. Making an apology was important to me, even if she didn't want to hear it. I did what I could forty years too late, and was rejected. I don't blame her for choosing not to speak with me.

Now that the dust has settled, I've had time to figure out what I learned from the experience. Here goes: I learned when you come to a fork in the road, and must decide which path to take, the long, painful, difficult path is the correct one. The fast, easy, convenient, path, is the wrong one. It's human nature to make things easy on ourselves, so, often as not, we take the wrong path. It was a difficult lesson and I went through hell to learn it. Like I said, I'm hard-headed. Today, I keep her picture next to my bed, as I have for forty years, because our time together brought the happiest moments of my life. We were just kids, but I've never been more happy. Now my story is told, but I still owe you six words. The End, and that's the truth.

Suggested Reading
About Stroke and
Traumatic Brain Injury

Over My Head by Dr. Claudia L. Osborn

I first read this book while in hospital recovering from my stroke. Dr. Osborn had many of the same problems from her brain injury as I did from stroke, so I was with her every step of the way. This is a very popular book within the medical community. An interesting read I'd recommend to others who want better understanding of the effects of traumatic brain injury.

My Stroke of Luck by Kirk Douglas

Someone in my stroke support group recommended I read this book. I did and I enjoyed it. I was surprised to learn Mr. Douglas came to the same conclusion about helping people as I have. I wish Mr. Douglas had told me how he arrived at that conclusion. I wonder if it was dogma or the result of personal experience. Interesting if you want to know more about Kirk Douglas. He's a good man and has had an interesting life.

SNAP SHOTS

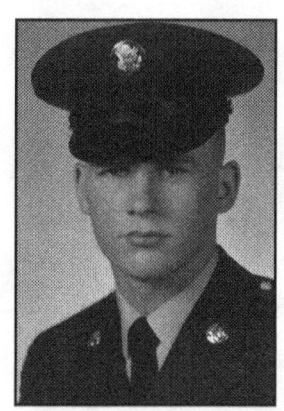

The author was 19 years old in 1966 at Ft. Gordon, Ga. prior to shipping out for the Republic of South Viet Nam where he served as a communications specialist and radioman with the Army Security Agency and served with the 337 Radio Research Company, 1st Infantry Division, for two years.

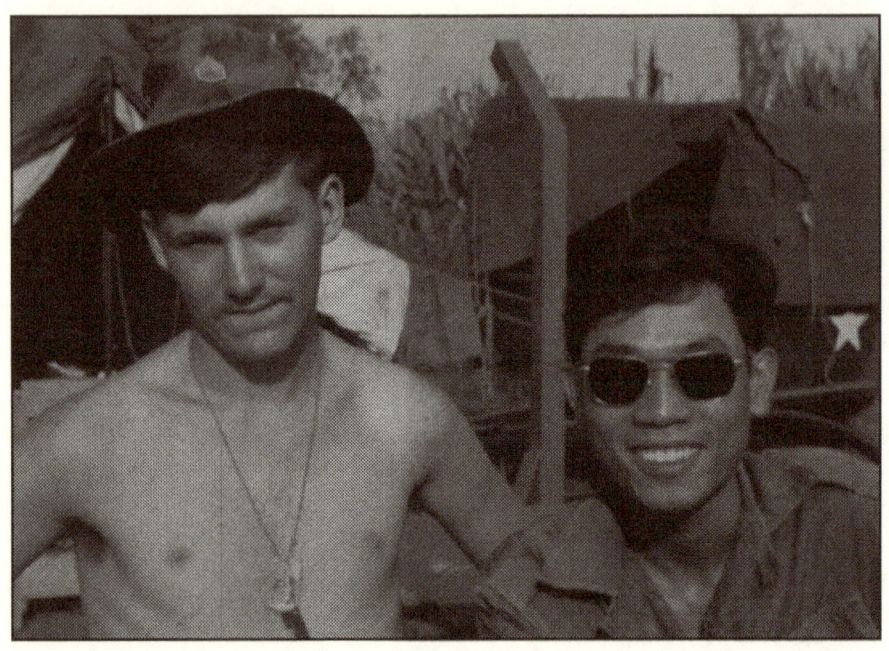

The author at 20 years of age with ARVN Sgt. Tran, the commo platoon interpreter, near An Loc RVN 1967. The author was wounded by friendly fire the following week. In 1969 he was promoted to Platoon Sergeant and awarded The Army Commendation Medal, The Good Conduct Medal, The National Defense Service Medal, The Viet Nam Service Medal, and The Viet Nam Campaign Medal for his service in the Republic of South Viet Nam. He later served with the 12th Special Forces.

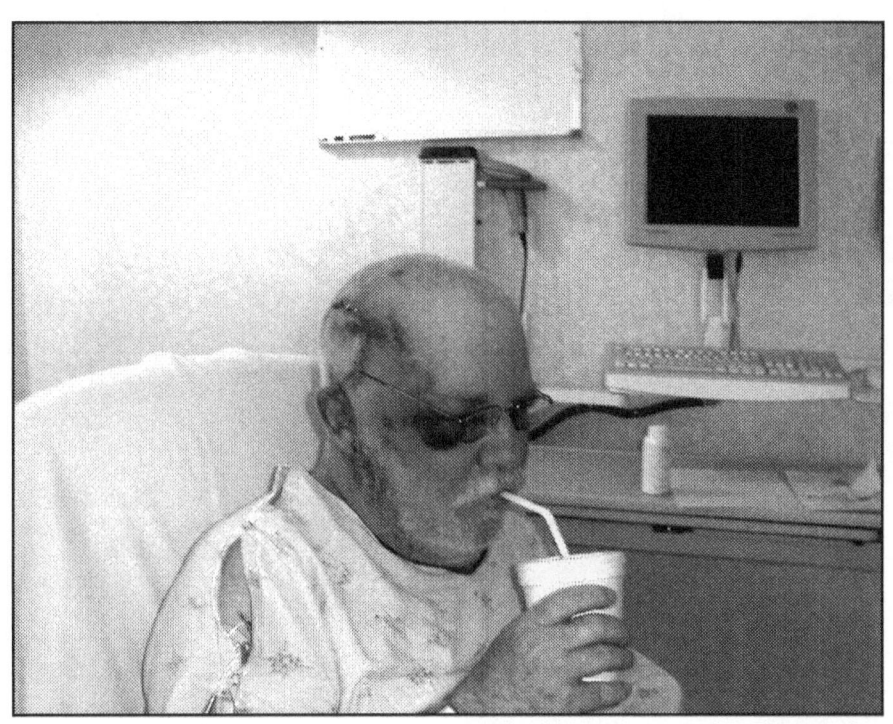

The author at 57 in 2004 following neurosurgery. The crescent shaped scar above his ear is where his brain was removed and replaced with sawdust and wood shavings.

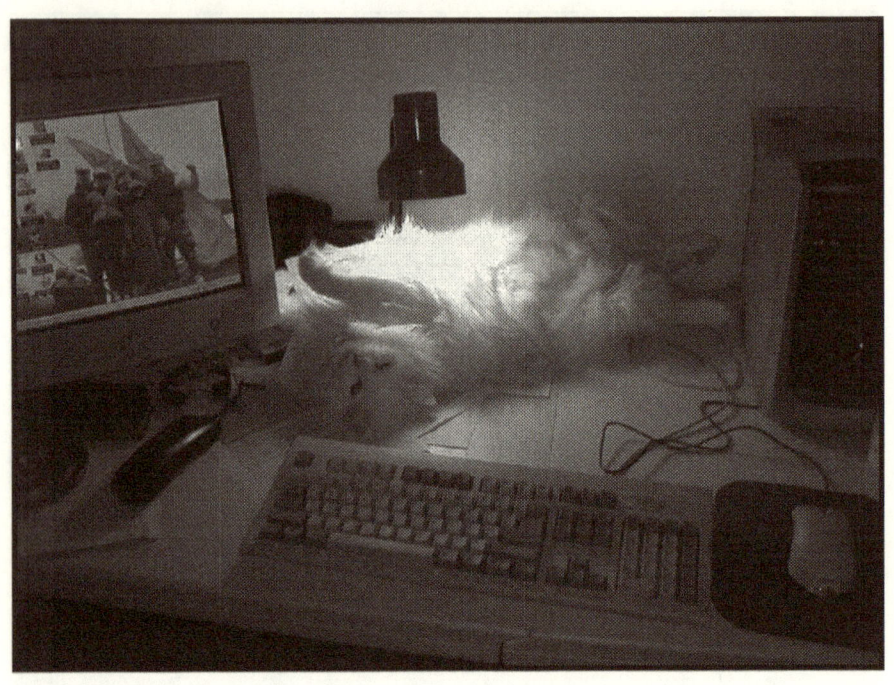

Kato, the author's Carolina bobbed-tail cat. Kato is a descendant of cats brought to the colonies by English settlers and sailors. She has helped the author from this "relaxed" position for eight years. She is definitely the brains of the outfit.

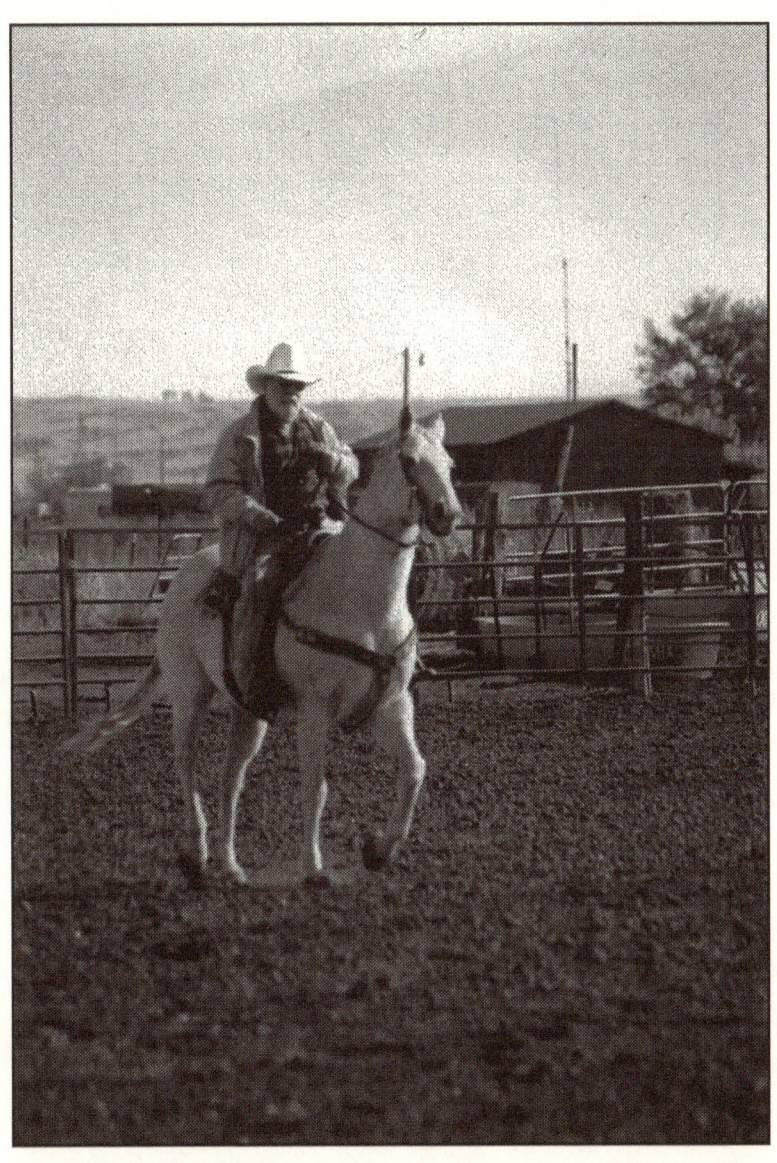

Back in the saddle in 2005. The Author at 58 stirs the tiller aboard Paycheck, a champion team-roping horse near Billings, Montana.

END NOTES

[1] American Stroke Association meeting Presentation

[2] American Heart Association data

[3] American Heart Association data

[4] American Stroke Association information

[5] National Center for Disease Control data

[6] Scientific American August 2005 issue p. 21,22

[7] Stroke Connection Magazine, Nov. Dec. 2004 Edition

[8] Stroke Connection Magazine, May-June 2005 Edition

[9] On Death and Dying by Dr. Elisabeth Kubler-Ross

[10] Lauren Bacall

[11] High Blood Pressure is a form of heart disease. One
in five Americans has it per NCHS

[12] American Stroke Association Data

[13] Data per Independent Sector

[14] Data per Johns Hopkins Medicine Office of Communications and Public Affairs

[15] Aldous Huxley, The Doors of Perception

[16] from Stroke Connection Magazine Nov./Dec. 2004

[17] Albert Camus. Translation by Justin O'Brien 1955

[18] American Stroke Association Data

www.ingramcontent.com/pod-product-compliance
Lightning Source LLC
Chambersburg PA
CBHW031951170526
45157CB00002B/459